McLachlan's Handbook of Diagnosis and Treatment of Venereal Diseases

McLachlan's Handbook of Diagnosis and Treatment of Venereal Diseases

---

A. S. Grimble
M.D., M.R.C.P.

Fifth Edition

E. & S. LIVINGSTONE LTD
EDINBURGH AND LONDON 1969

SBN 443 00653 9

Printed in Great Britain

Preface to Fifth Edition

The venereal diseases no longer exist as a group of conditions of which the medical profession is unmindful, nor do they form too delicate a subject for public discussion. The last decade has not only seen these disorders strengthen their hold on most communities in the world, but witnessed a renewal of public and professional concern about their prevalence. Today there is a healthy interest in their existence, treatment and control. As the world 'grows smaller' so the likelihood remains that these diseases will persist in human communities everywhere.

Although it is not always in the interest of a lay person to know too much about certain diseases which may breed anxiety, it is necessary for some of the facts to be appreciated by all persons above the age of puberty. McLachlan's Handbook contained, in its original author's hands, a succinct account of the principle diseases. The matter was set out most readably and the subject thoroughly covered and accompanied by many illustrations, which greatly added to the interest and assisted readers without special experience of the venereal diseases. It is to be hoped that the standard has been maintained, and also its usefulness whether to doctors, students or nurses.

The sexually transmitted diseases are to be considered more as a group of lower genito-urinary inflammations related to sexuality, rather than in the narrower sense of one or two disorders with sexual promiscuity as their *raison d'être*. In the present edition the introductory and general descriptive chapters on those on techniques are accompanied by other short sections on closely related subjects. This has widened the field of discussion without increasing the size of the volume.

Acknowledgements

The sincere gratitude of the editor is due to Miss Anne Becher for the typing of the script, to Dr. George Rohatiner for his care and suggestions when reading the script, to the publishers for their helpfulness and also in this respect to Mrs. McLachlan.

Acknowledgements and thanks for certain of the illustrations and the figures used in the graphs are due to Guy's Hospital Medical School Departments of Photography and Medical Illustration and the Photographic Unit of the Interdepartmental Laboratory, Dr. G. Csonka, Dr. E. Dunlop, Dr. I. Harper, Dr. E. Klieneberger-Nobel, Dr. A. Tinkler, Dr. A. Wilkinson, The Home Office, and May and Baker Ltd.

1969 A. S. G.

Contents

ERRATA

Page 4. The caption to figures 5A and B should read as follows:

Candida albicans, showing mainly yeasts in specimen (A) and mainly hyphae in specimen (B). Gram staining.

Page 45. The 8th line from the bottom should read as follows:

The serum tests are not commonly negative in the presence. . . .

Page 98. The legend to figure 102 should read as follows:

Chancroidal ulceration of preputial meatus, showing typical 'fuzzy' appearance.

The legend to figure 103 should read as follows:

Chancroid of corona glandis, and fluctuating bubo.

Page 118. The 4th line from the bottom should read as follows:

days, is useful, and kanamycin and Septrin may also be. . . .

Page 175. In the legend to figure 154 the word corneal should be altered to coronal.

CHAPTER 1

Introduction

The study of venereal diseases is concerned with the infective and non-infective lesions, usually inflammatory, which are *sexually transmitted*. A few of these infective diseases are endemic in almost every part of the world. Some of them, notably syphilis, have become sporadic in certain countries. But there is still a tendency for small epidemics of a venereal disease to arise in any country during periods of social unrest, war or instability.

In recent years the use of antibiotics, along with higher living standards and general increase in health, has had a marked effect on the clinical features of some of these diseases. Venereal disease must be seen in its social setting, in relation to society and its customs as well as to individuals, their attitudes and their behaviour. Epidemiological problems occur in connection with the infectious carrier, sexual promiscuity, perversion, prostitution, homosexuality, and in relation to the law.

In Britain the law has recognised for its own purposes only three infections as 'venereal', by definition; whereas the speciality is, in fact, one concerned more widely in its clinical aspects with lower genito-urinary medicine.

The effects of sexually transmitted disorders form a part of the professional experience of all practitioners of medicine and are as likely to be seen in other general or specialist clinics as in venereology.

MICROBIOLOGY

Although many different micro-organisms or parasites may be transferred from person to person during sexual intercourse, only those commonly transferred in this manner can be said to be venereal. The more usual ones are shown in Table 1.

Chlamydia oculogenitale (TRIC virus agent)

This virus is a member of a group also known as *Bedsoniae*, and its presence is demonstrated by initial bodies and inclusion bodies in the cytoplasm of epithelial cells. The virus can be grown on embryonated eggs from the sites of infection: conjunctiva, urethra and cervix. The initial or elementary body (infective particle) is 0.2–0.4 μ in diameter.

TABLE 1

Virus:	*Chlamydia oculogenitale* (TRIC virus), *Lymphogranuloma venereum.*
Mycoplasma:	*M. hominis* } variable parasitism. 'T' strain }
Donovan body:	*Donovania granulomatis.*
Bacteria:	*Haemophilus ducreyi, Neisseria gonorrhoeae.* Other bacteria: *E. coli,* streptococci, staphylococci.
Spirochaete:	*Treponema pallidum.*
Yeast-like:	*Candida albicans* (and others).
Protozoon:	*Trichomonas vaginalis.*

Lymphpgranuloma venereum

This virus also belongs to the group *Bedsoniae*, which, unlike true viruses, possess both DNA and RNA. Visible inclusion bodies appear in mononuclear cells, and the organism may be propagated in tissue culture and chick embryo. The virus is transmitted by sexual intercourse; it has a world-wide distribution and it can exist in a population group without causing disease symptoms. It has been shown in a survey in east London, where the case incidence was 2 per cent, that 14 per cent of patients possessed serum complement fixing antibodies in borderline titres. Usually it causes a local genital lesion, bubo, and occasionally a general relapsing illness.

Mycoplasma

These organisms, which in their metabolic activity lie nearer to the bacteria than the viruses, have no true cell membrane. Their minimal reproductive units are only 125 mμ in size and will therefore pass through bacterial filters. Mycoplasma occurs widely in nature both as a saprophyte and as a parasite. In diseases undoubtedly caused by these organisms, as for example in atypical pneumonia in man, and in animal diseases, it is not entirely clear how the infection occurs. The more parasitic strains of organism are fastidious in their requirements for cultivation in cell-free media. Mycoplasma is found in the mouth

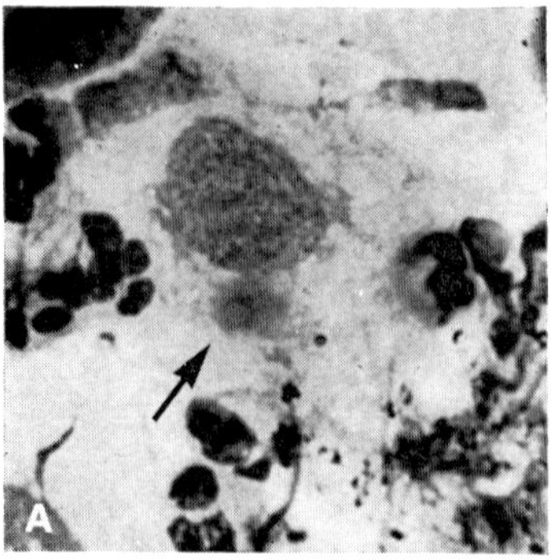

FIG. 1.

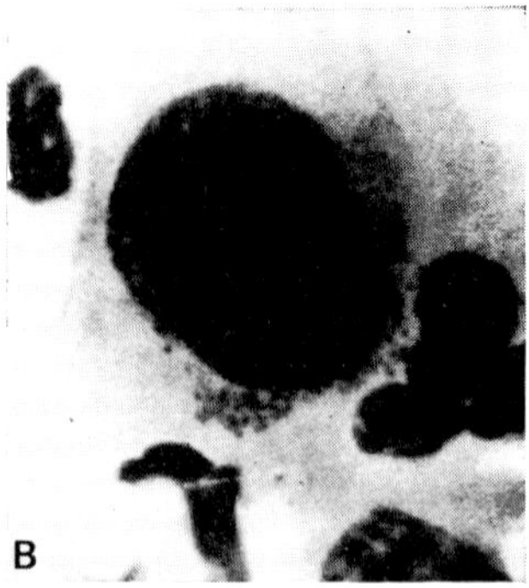

FIG. 2

Chlamydia oculogenitale: (*a*) initial body in cytoplasm of epithelial cell. Giemsa staining. (*b*) elementary bodies in cytoplasm around nucleus of epithelial cell. Giemsa staining.

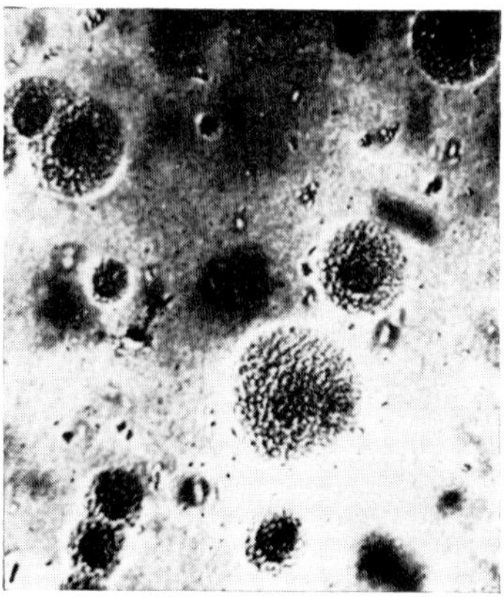

FIG. 3.

Mycoplasma colonies on enriched agar: *M. hominis*.

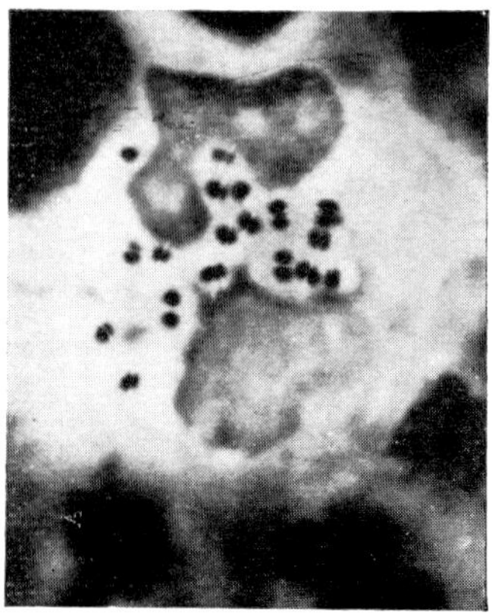

FIG. 4.

Neisseria gonorrhoeae: kidney-shaped pairs of cocci lying in cytoplasm of the leucocyte. ($\times$ 975) Gram staining.

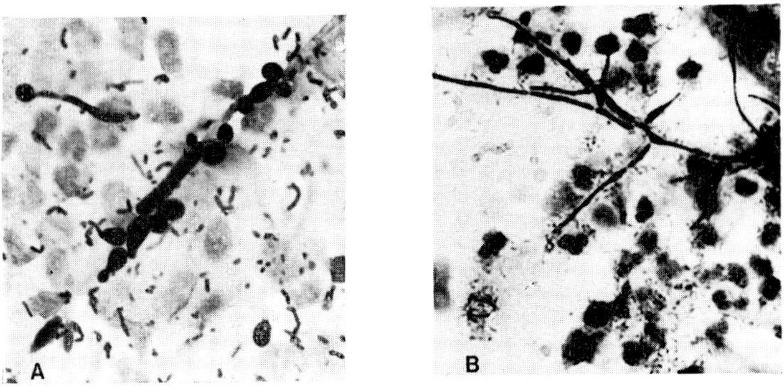

FIG. 5.

Candida albicans, showing mainly hyphae in specimen (*a*) and mainly yeasts in (*b*). Gram staining.

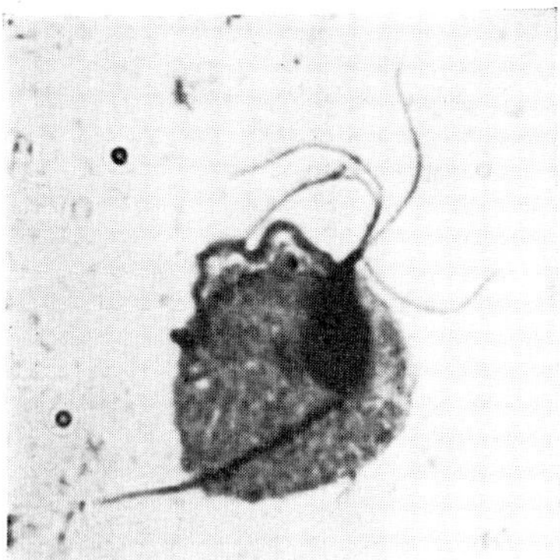

FIG. 6.

Trichomonas vaginalis as seen in a wet film; the flagellae and membrane are caught in rapid movement.

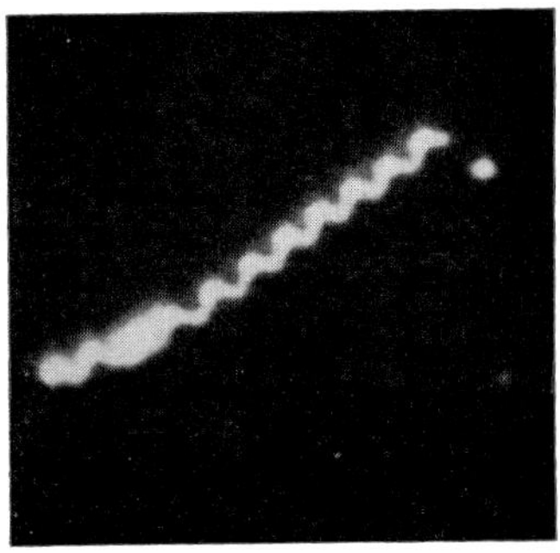

FIG. 7.

Treponema pallidum as seen on dark-ground microscopy.

and respiratory tract, but the commonest site of the organism is the genital tract, and genital infection would presumably therefore be not unexpected. Isolations of mycoplasma have been made from various genital and pelvic abscesses and also from abacterial puerperal septicaemia. Yet the problem of genital infection with mycoplasma remains largely unsolved; there are several factors that tend to 'light up' an infection which would otherwise be less likely or unlikely to occur. The genital organisms exist in two strains: the hominis (three types) and the 'T' (tiny) strain.

Donovan body (*D. granulomatis*)

This is a parasitic organism (probably protozoon) found especially in the large mononuclear leucocytes in the blood or lesions of the disease granuloma inguinale. It occurs only in man, causing genital ulcerations or more general infection.

Haemophilus ducreyi

This is a small Gram-negative bacillus 1·5 μ in diameter which causes chancroid. The bacilli are often seen in clusters or chains, are non-motile and non-sporing, and are difficult to culture, requiring the addition of blood to the medium. The organism is not usually of high virulence; it is seen more frequently in warm climates, infection resulting in local genital lesions only.

Neisseria gonorrhoeae

These are Gram-negative, kidney-shaped diplococci, with flat surfaces opposed, and measure less than 1 μ in diameter. There are several commensal, as well as one other pathogenic member of the group *Neisseria*. It is a strictly human parasite resulting in genital discharge. The disease was well known in antiquity. Hydrocoele fluid, blood or serum must be added to the growth medium; most strains will grow better in an atmosphere containing 5 per cent carbon dioxide.

Treponema pallidum

This is a spirochaete varying in length, but on average 7–12 μ; long and short forms occur. The typically regular spirals (or waves) number between 6 and 14. Granules, round bodies and various morphological alterations occur as a result of growth under adverse conditions. The importance of a granular stage, apart from its very small size, is the possible diminution in susceptibility to inhibitory substances (*e.g.*, antibiotics) which it implies. The organism cannot be grown in cell-free culture, and most of the studies on the *Treponema pallidum* have been performed using techniques of animal inoculation. Infection can result in the chronic, serious, possibly life-long disease of syphilis.

Candida albicans (and other species of *Candida*)

These yeast-like organisms are not uncommonly present in moist areas of the body including the genital tract. They may be seen as 'spores' (or oval yeast cells), as mycelia, or as globular, thick-walled chlamydo-spores. *Candida albicans* may be found either with or without inflammatory changes in the epithelium; other species are also implicated in genital infection.

Trichomonas vaginalis

This is an inhabitant of the genito-urinary tract. It is a pear-shaped protozoon, 9–15 μ long, with nucleus and cytostome, undulating membrane projecting over the posterior end, and three to five flagella very active from the broad end when viewed in wet-preparation, preferably under dark-ground microscopy. A similar protozoon, *T. hominis*, is found in the alimentary tract, particularly in the tropics.

Since man is unique amongst animals in his sexual responsiveness, disorders may be expected to arise from time to time from this activity, be it marital, premarital or extramarital. The changing attitudes to this subject are reflected in the increasing numbers of enquiries made by patients attending clinics with conditions centred in their minds on their sexual activity.

The overall pattern of these diseases is not static, and can be expected to continue to change. Although syphilis will remain sporadic, if not endemic, there is little doubt that the severe lesions of late syphilis will be seen less frequently in communities where individuals freely obtain antibiotics. This places a greater responsibility on the laboratory tests used to detect syphilitic antibodies and on judicious performance of these tests in the absence of clinical signs. So far as we know, no treponemal resistance has yet arisen to antibiotics at present in use. However, today, higher doses of antibiotic are considered essential than two decades ago.

Ulcerative and papular lesions of the genitalia are commonly secondary to infective causes within the lower genital tract, or due to such lesions as herpes simplex, thrush or scabies. Chancroid, and the conditions discussed along with it in Chapter 6, are becoming more uncommon. Their importance lies in the need to exclude syphilis.

The cause of urethritis, vaginitis or cervicitis cannot always be determined. Consideration must be given to such factors as traumatic, irritative, allergic, primary or secondary infection. It is often possible to make an aetiological diagnosis, or at least an assessment of the probable cause, only after both partners have been seen and examined. The incidence of these inflammations shows no signs of diminishing.

In the British Isles, abacterial urethritis in men occurs more frequently than gonorrhoea; many of the abacterial infections are seen in stable sexual couples. As an illustration: in 25 cases of rheumatism and arthritis following urethritis in men the sexual background was as follows: wife or fiancee or close friend, 13 cases; coitus with prostitute or stranger, nine cases; with an acquaintance, three cases.

PRINCIPAL DAMAGING EFFECTS

The inflammation resulting from sexually transmitted infection varies greatly in severity and extent. The potentially most damaging disease is syphilis. Unless treated, this is frequently a life-long disease, and may also infect the foetus *in utero*. Other infections presenting as 'sores', which include chancroid, granuloma inguinale and lymphogranuloma venereum, result as a rule in few complications.

Any infectious discharge from the genital tract may proceed to a variety of complications, local and general, mild or severe. In women, gonorrhoea is the most dangerous of the possible causes of such an inflammation. However, in men, so far as is known, similar complications may result from an infection with any one of several pathogenic micro-organisms. The principal disorders which occur are inflammations of the pelvic organs and tissues and their sequelae, or rheumatism and arthritis.

In women the occurrence of *carcinoma of the cervix* has been shown to be connected with coitus, having an increased frequency where there is an early onset of sexual intercourse and where the individual remarries in later life.

DEFINITION OF 'VENEREAL'

Lower genito-urinary infection resulting in a discharge may be due to a variety of agencies. When such a discharge is due to a micro-organism which has its existence *primarily* in the genital epithelium, then that infection is rarely transmitted except by sexual intercourse; and for the appearance of such a disorder (for example gonorrhoea) intercourse would have to have taken place with an *already infected person* who themselves had contracted the disease in the same way. On the other hand, where the organism might possibly exist also in other sites, although usually transmitted by sexual intercourse, coitus with an already infected person is *not* essential. Both conditions are strictly 'venereal'.

The diseases described in Part 1 are almost always sexually transmitted: other conditions, however, described in Part 3, are met with in both a 'venereal' and a 'non-venereal' context; that is, they are met with as sexually transmitted disorders, and as infections arising in other ways. The disorders commonly seen in the clinic, which are closely related to sexual transmission, are gonorrhoea, trichomoniasis, condylomata acuminata, and possibly TRIC virus and mycoplasma infection. Other genital conditions often sexually transmitted are candidasis, herpes simplex progenitalis, scabies and phthiriasis. The expression 'sexually transmitted disorder', being less weighted with moral overtones, would seem to be more acceptable to both medical practitioners and the general public than the older term 'venereal'.

SUGGESTED READING

Morton, R. S. (1966). *Introduction to Venereal Diseases*. Harmondsworth: Penguin Books.

PART 1

Syphilis and Venereal Sores

CHAPTER 2

Early Infectious Syphilis (Primary Syphilis) — Chancre.

INTRODUCTION

Syphilis is a contagious disease caused by the *Treponema pallidum*, which, after penetration of the skin or mucous surface, causes a local sore whilst it gradually invades every organ and tissue of the body, with subsequent liability to early or later manifestations of the disease in any of these structures. The organism can infect *without* the appearance of a local lesion.

Syphilis may be acquired by direct or mediate contact, and *in utero*. Direct infection in almost all cases is by sexual contact, and less commonly by perversions or kissing. Digital contact may result in local infection. *Mediate* infection has occurred, from imperfectly cleansed eating or drinking utensils, especially cracked or chipped ones, or from the common use of toilet articles and professional or industrial instruments. Such cases are now unknown. Blood transfusion has been responsible for a number of infections. Invasion via the placental capillaries is known as *congenital syphilis*.

REINFECTION

The reinfection of a fully treated original infection with syphilis results in the usual features of clinical syphilis (or their absence). Reinfection of an *already infected* individual results in a modified clinical picture.

COURSE OF SEXUALLY ACQUIRED SYPHILIS

The course of untreated acquired syphilis has, for many years, been divided on clinical grounds into primary, secondary and tertiary stages. A better classification is into *early infectious syphilis*, comprising the primary and secondary stages, together with early asymptomatic infection and *late syphilis*, including all manifestations occurring more than two years after infection. The stages may be summarised as in Table 2.

IMMUNE RESPONSE TO SYPHILIS

Man possesses no natural immunity to syphilis. It is clear, however, both on clinical grounds and from the results of experiments undertaken on human volunteers, that acquired immunity develops; and from animal studies it would appear that this immunity is of both the cellular and the humoral kind.

TABLE 2

COURSE OF UNTREATED SYPHILIS (VERY APPROXIMATE)

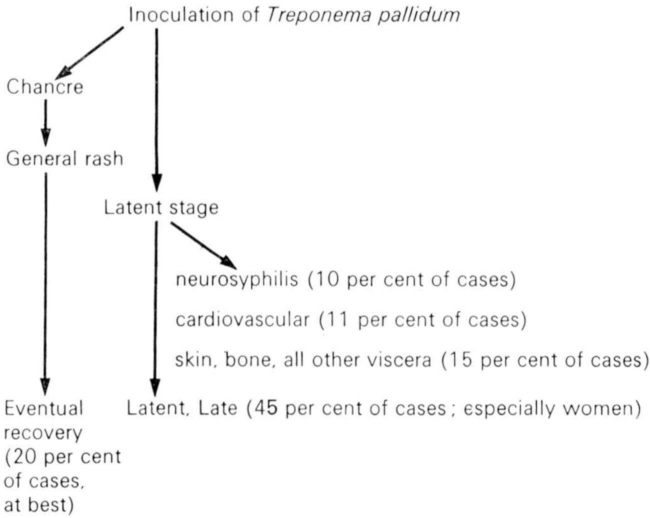

The manner in which the body reacts to the treponeme determines the type of lesion, in developed syphilis the important factors being the presence of circulating antibody and tissue hypersensitivity.

In recent years the *Treponema pallidum* has been isolated from syphilitic patients who have received standard amounts of antibiotic treatment. These isolations have been made with the greatest facility from the eye and the central nervous system.

Moreover some of these have occurred in patients who did not have any circulating antibodies (*i.e.*, had negative serum tests).

Chancre

It must be remembered that the course of syphilis does not invariably run true to type. The primary sore may be trivial and unnoticed, or may be absent (syphilis *d'emblée*). Thus in the investigation of a patient presenting with a general rash there may be no history or no clinical evidence, on searching examination, of a primary sore, while patients in the late stages may deny, in all good faith, knowledge of any antecedent sore or subsequent skin rash. In certain of these cases, in males, the history of urethral discharge may suggest the possible date of an unrecognised intraurethral chancre or anal chancre.

CHARACTERISTICS

Following an incubation period of about two to four weeks, but usually three (wide variations are rare), the primary sore appears at the site of inoculation. Constitutional disturbances, such as malaise, headache, pains in the joints, anaemia and pyrexia, can occur at this stage, more especially in women.

Beginning as a dusky red macule, the chancre presents as, (1) an erosion or fissure, (2) an ulceration or (3) a papule which subsequently undergoes superficial erosion or deeper ulceration. Infrequently the appearance is that of a dry scaly papule. The characteristics of the primary sore are: (*a*) It is generally *single*; a few cases show multiple sores; if multiple all the lesions show the same age characteristics. (*b*) The sore is *round* or *ovoid* with a greyish or dusky red granulomatous or sloughy base. Crusting may occur. (*c*) The sore is *painless*, and does not bleed freely—a slight initial bleeding after cleansing is rapidly followed by an ooze of clear serum in which *T. pallidum* can be demonstrated, unless lotions or creams have been applied locally. (*d*) In over 50 per cent of cases the lesion is surrounded by a well-defined dusky-pink areola 1 mm.–2 mm. broad. (*e*) The serum tests for syphilis at this stage are generally negative. (*f*) *Induration*,

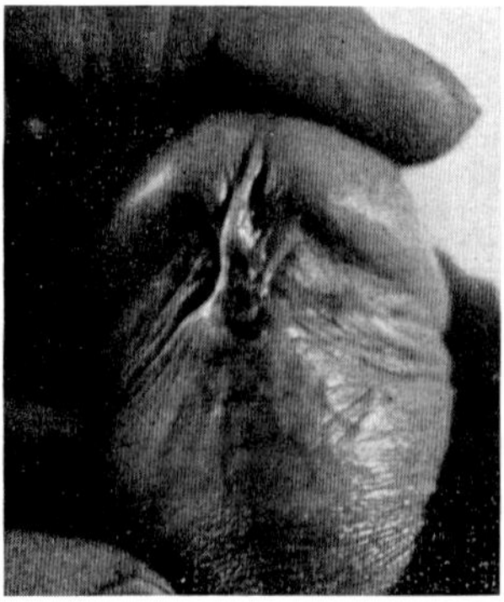

FIG. 8.

Early primary sore of frenum; no areola, no induration.

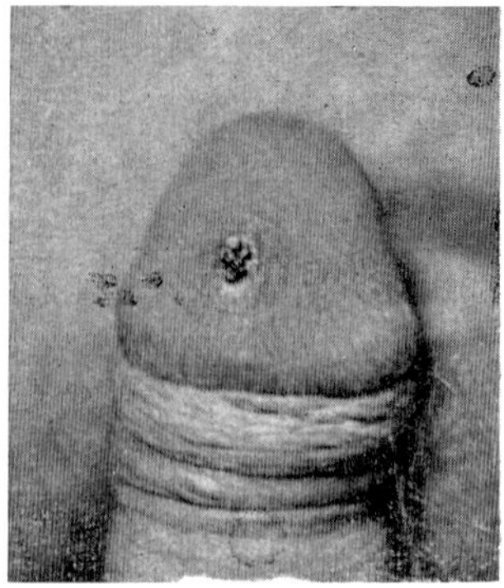

FIG. 9.

Early ulcerative primary sore of glans penis; areola and induration absent.

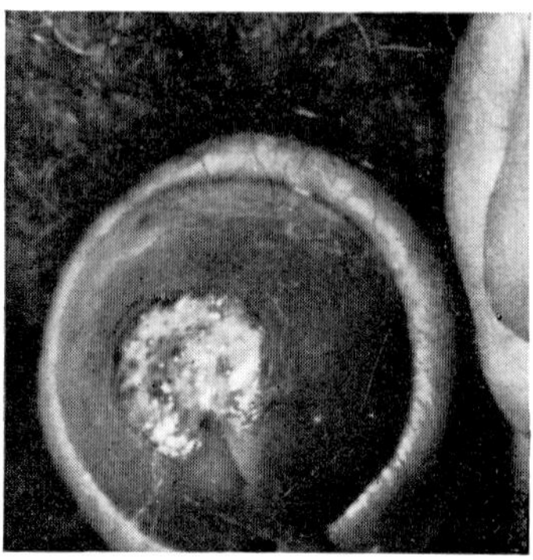

FIG. 10.

Meatal chancre of erosive type.

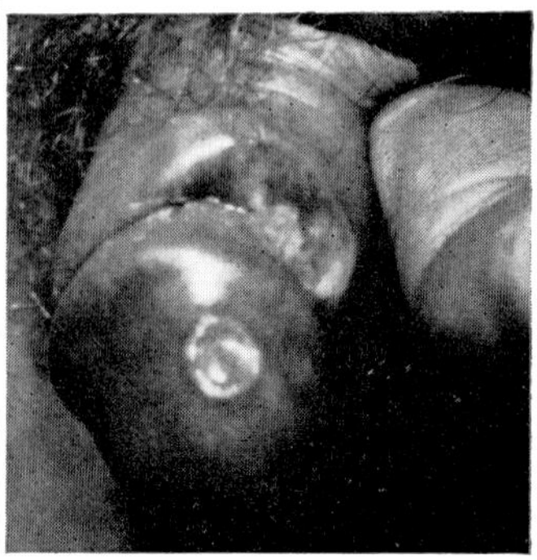

FIG. 11.

Chancre of sulcus with indurated rim; 'kissing chancre' on glans.

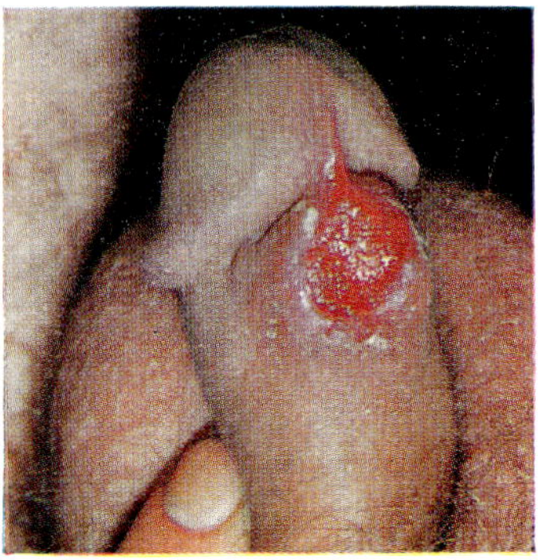

FIG. 12.

Indurated chancre of frenum.

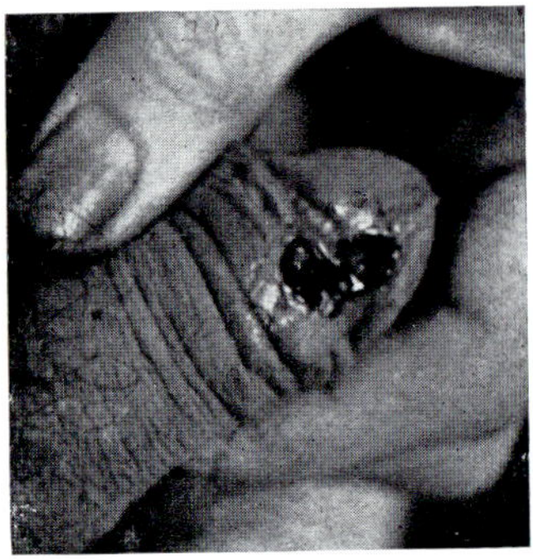

FIG. 13.

Crusted primary sore at site of torn frenum.

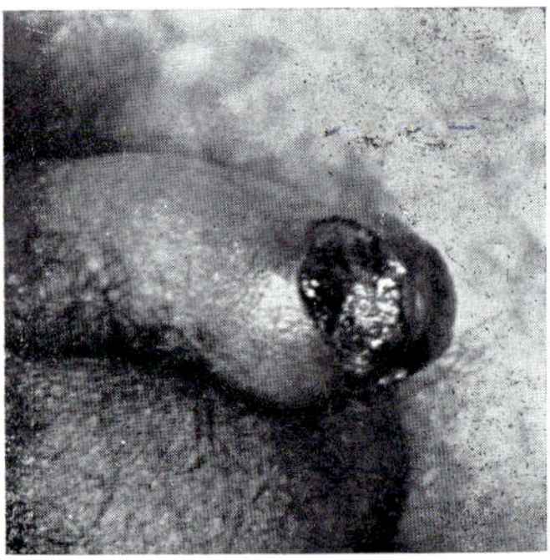

FIG. 14.

Granulomatous primary sore on outer aspect of prepuce.

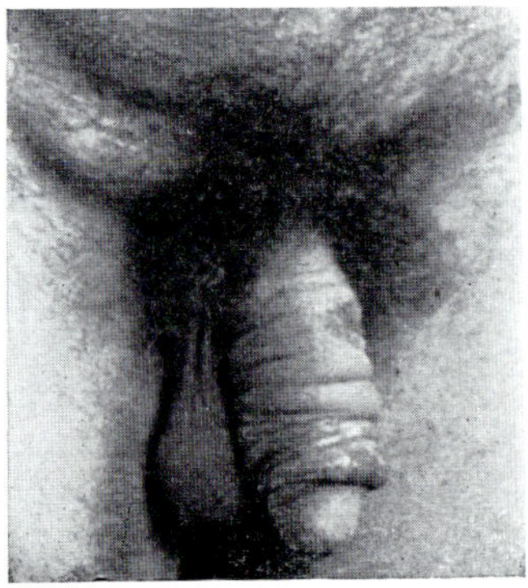

FIG. 15.

Granulomatous sore on shaft of the penis; lymphangitis and marked inguinal adenitis.

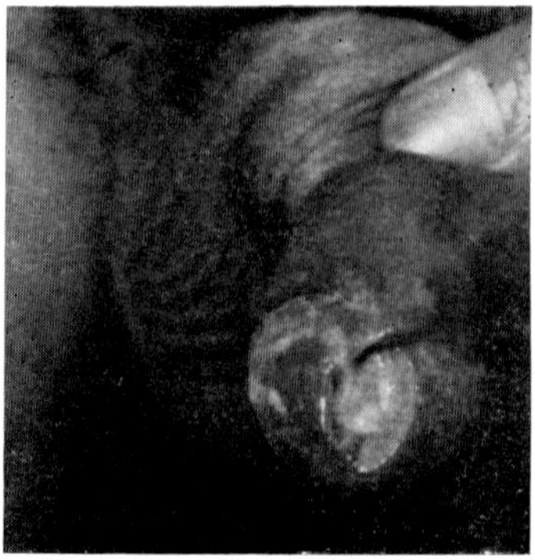

FIG. 16.

Ulceration with excavation due to chancre of frenum.

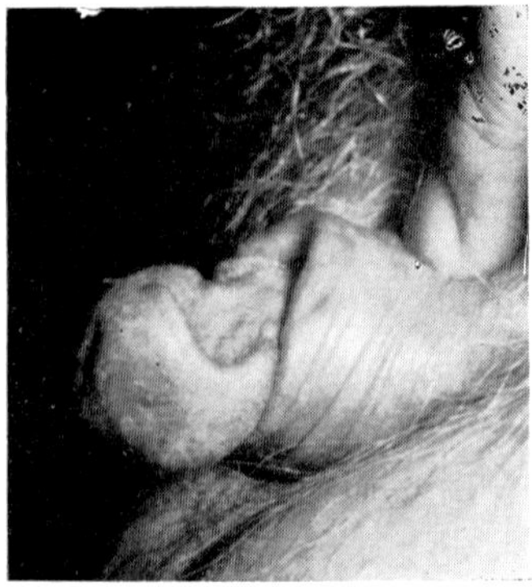

FIG 17.

Healed chancre showing destruction of frenum.

affecting first the edges of the sore and comparable to the raised rim of a coat button, later involves the whole base of the sore and gradually extends beyond its limits into the surrounding tissues, giving rise to a feeling of elastic cartilaginous hardness (a typical Hunterian chancre). (*g*) *Regional adenitis*—a painless, discrete, elastic, globoid swelling of the regional lymph glands, occurs early. Later, rarely, there may be brawny, painless, indolent lymphangitis, the colour of the overlying skin varying from normal to a dusky-pink. *T. pallidum* is demonstrable in the exudate of the sore and in the gland aspirate (p. 21). The primary sore varies from a diameter of 0·2 cm.–3 cm. or more. There are no significant differences in the two sexes, but important variations, due principally to the site of the lesion, must be borne in mind. In men half of all chancres are subpreputial, and oedema and lymphangitis may lead to phimosis. Secondary pyogenic infection is not uncommon beneath the non-retractable prepuce and it may convert the lesion into a painful ragged ulcer. The subpreputial discharge may be either thin or purulent, and in the latter instance the demonstration of the *T. pallidum* is difficult. Exposure of the sore by dorsal or lateral slitting of the prepuce may be necessary. Diagnosis can be effected by demonstrating the *T. pallidum* in the juice obtained by gland puncture, if not from the lesion itself.

Other variations to be remembered are chancres of the *preputial meatus*, which are sometimes multiple and often seemingly trivial fissures, mistaken for traumatic lesions. Chancres of the *meatus* may present as typical circummeatal erosions: scanty urethral discharge and dysuria may suggest urethritis. Suspicion should also be aroused by a unilateral oedema or induration of the epithelium of the glans. On the *shaft* of the penis the sore may be more crusted, with less induration in the early stages. In the *anus* it may be fissured.

In women, chancres of the *cervix uteri* are commonest, are usually single, and in appearance are erosive, not uncommonly papuloulcerative, infrequently hypertrophic and fungating, or diffusely indurative. They are usually situated around the external os and may extend into the cervical canal. Solitary lesions seldom reach more than 2 cm. in diameter. The erosive type is dusky purplish red, contrasting with the brighter red of acute cervical infection and the pinker colour of chronic erosion. The margin is well defined as a rule with a marked dull areola. A false membrane sometimes covers the lesion and removal of this membrane is followed by some bleeding. Occasionally the chancre may lie within the cervical canal, in some cases resulting in an indurative oedema of the entire cervix.

The lymph drainage of the cervix is to the common iliac and mesorectal group of glands, and that of the upper vagina is to the inguinal group. On the labia majora and minora, and in the region of the fourchette, typical chancrous erosions or ulcerations are the rule. They may, however, be trivial in size or present as fissures. The prominent, brawny unilateral oedema of the entire labium should direct attention to the possibility of a chancre: in such a case inguinal adenitis is present.

EXTRAGENITAL CHANCRE

The commonest locations for chancre outside the genital area are the lip, tongue, tonsil, nipple and finger. On the *lip* the lesion

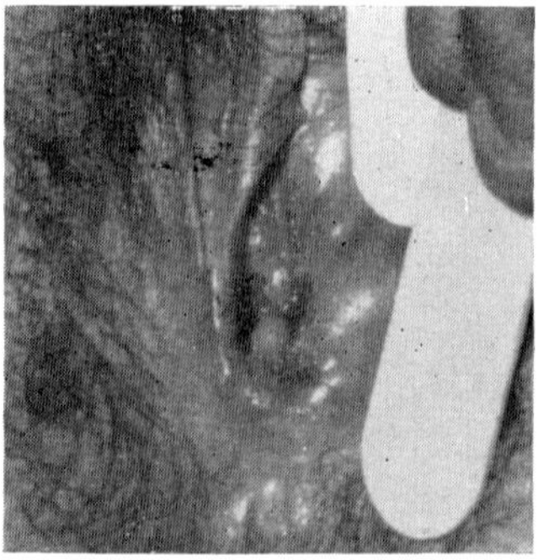

FIG. 18.

Chancre fissure near fourchette (*T. pallidum* +).

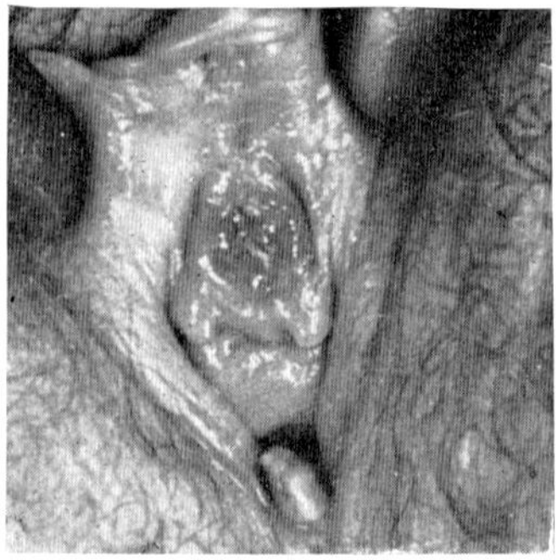

FIG. 19.

Areolated, erosive primary sore of female urethral orifice, with early induration.

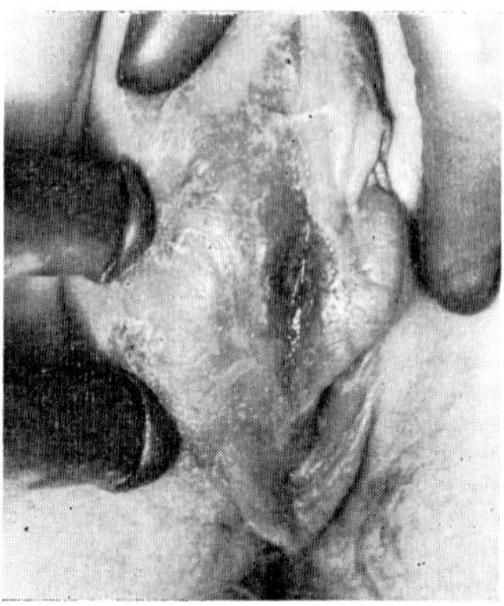

FIG. 20.

Primary sore in angle between right labium majus and minus; early 'bottom-rim' induration (*T. pallidum* +, W. R. negative).

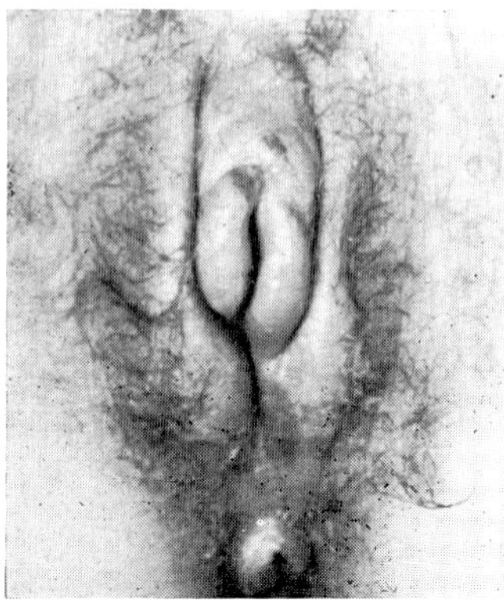

FIG. 21.

Small primary sore in the angle of the clitoris and labium minus, showing distribution of lymphangitic oedema.

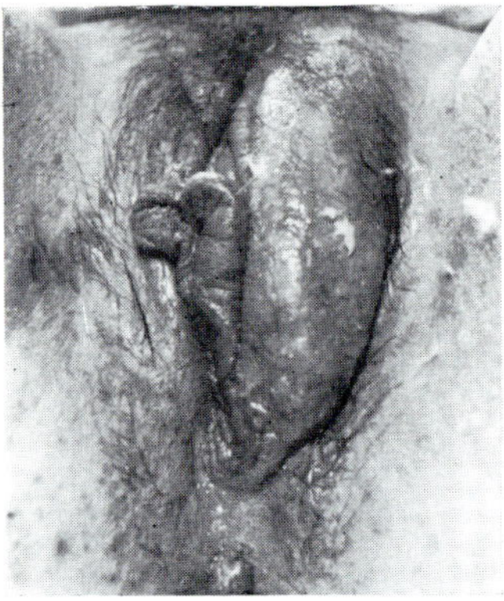

FIG. 22.

Marked labial oedema associated with primary sores. A skin rash is present.

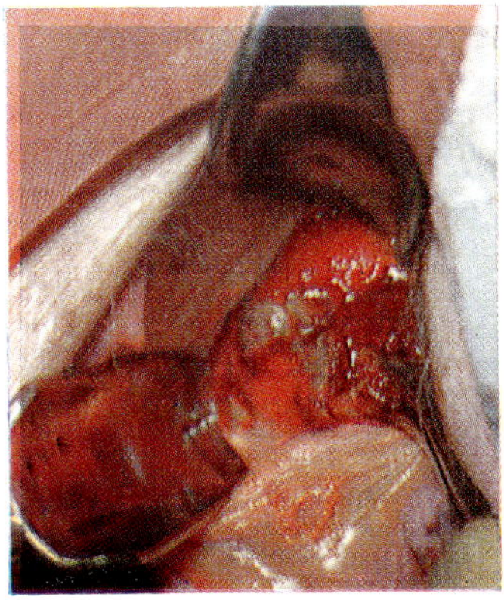

FIG. 23.

Chancre of cervix ; indurated, eroded, and dull red in colour.

is usually close to the midline and often passes as a 'cigarette burn'. Apposition or multiple chancres on the lips may occur. The lesion on the *tongue* is usually single and is seen near the tip, on the dorsum as a rule, with enlargement of the submental or submaxillary glands. The tongue therefore may not be freely moveable. When on the *tonsil* the lesion is commoner on the right than the left. Pain and sore throat may be present, pain being an unusual feature of syphilitic chancre in any position. The tonsil is enlarged and of a dusky red appearance, with ulceration and later pseudomembrane formation.

On the *nipple* and the surface of the finger, a chancre presents the usual appearance. But a lesion occurring in the *nail-fold* simulates a subacute painful onychia or paronychia, with typical lymph node swelling in the drainage areas.

PATHOLOGICAL HISTOLOGY OF THE CHANCRE

The underlying pathological changes consist of capillary dilatation, swelling and proliferation of the endothelium, formation of new capillaries, perivascular infiltration with small round and plasma cells, and the formation of new fibrous tissue. The lumen of the vessels tends to become obliterated—stage of erosion or early ulceration of sore. The changes are at first localised and affect chiefly the capillaries, but later endarteritis and periarteritis of the larger vessels occur. The cellular infiltration and formation of fibrous tissue gradually extend throughout and beyond the limits of the sore. Giant cell formation may occur—stage of induration.

DIFFERENTIAL DIAGNOSIS

In the genital region the chancre must be differentiated from a lesion of the general rash (secondary) stage or of the late stage of syphilis, from chancroid, granuloma inguinale, lymphogranuloma, herpes simplex, from ulcerations following pyogenic infection, balanoposthitis, skin diseases such as psoriasis, lichen, scabies, carcinoma, non-specific ulcerations, and in addition, in women, from ulcerations occurring in thrush, trichomonas infection, and the Lipschütz and Behçet types of ulceration.

On the lip and tongue it is essential to exclude herpes simplex, thrush, certain skin diseases, tuberculosis, later forms of syphilis,

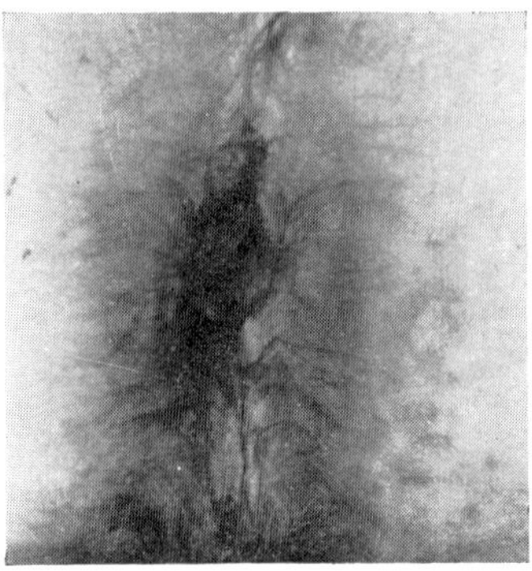

FIG. 24.

Primary sore presenting as an anal fissure at '12 o'clock'; an early rash is also present.

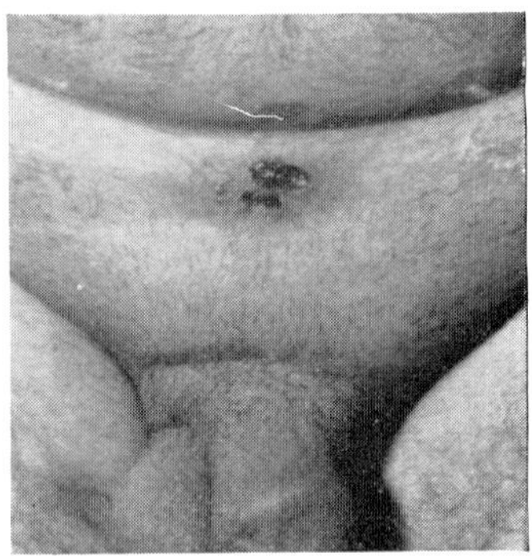

FIG. 25.

Chancre on lower abdomen.

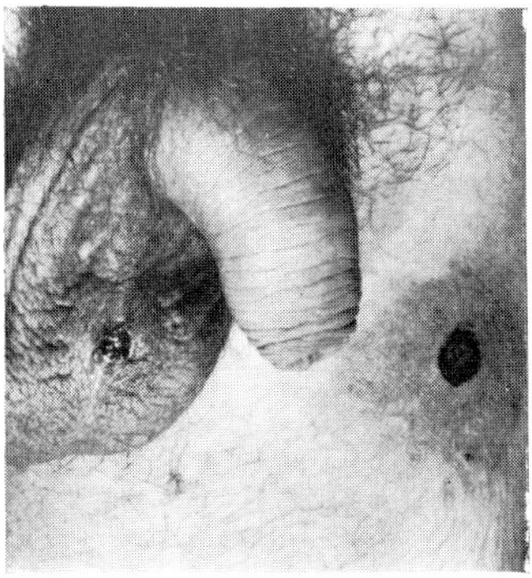

FIG. 26.

Primary sore of scrotal raphe and anterior surface of left thigh (*T. pallidum* +).

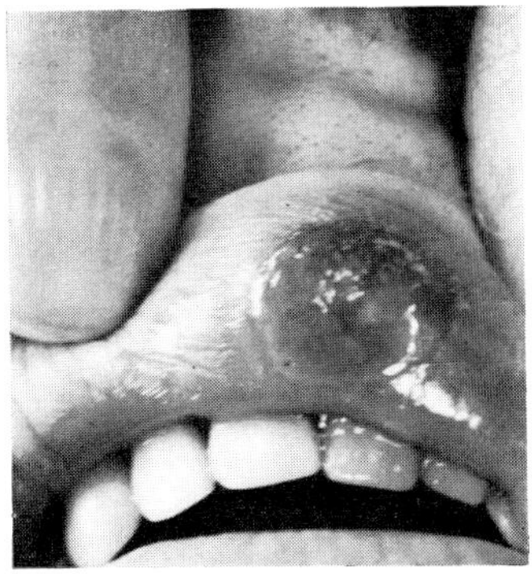

FIG. 27.

Areolated, erosive primary sore in centre of upper lip.

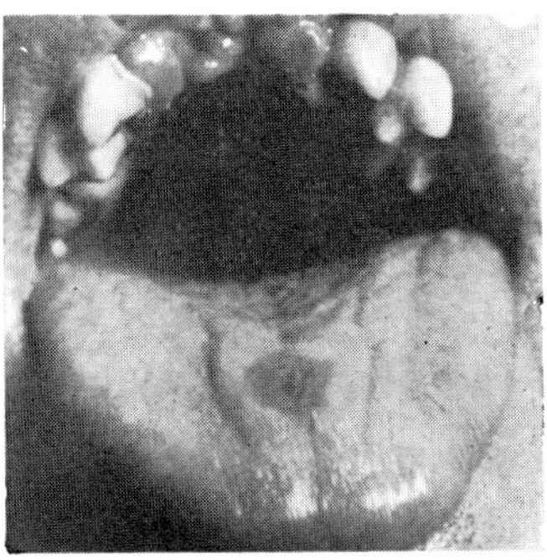

FIG. 28.

Primary sore of dorsum of the tongue.

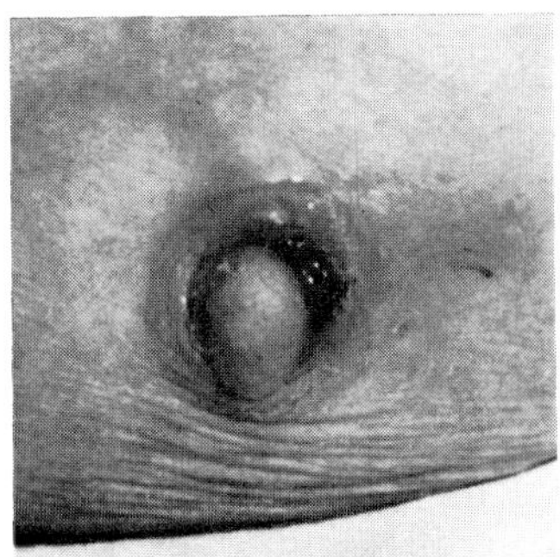

FIG. 29.

Primary sore of nipple.

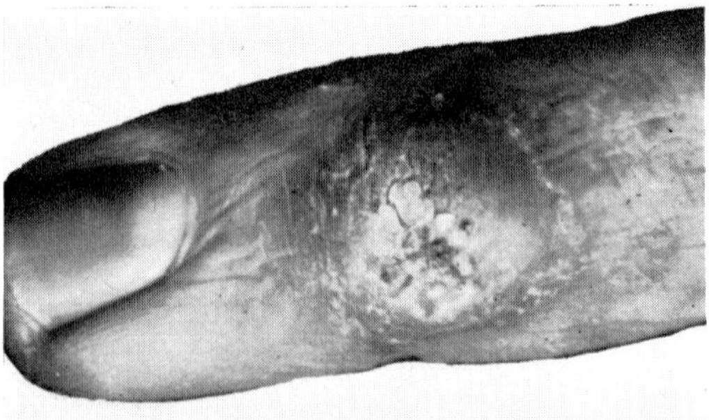

FIG. 30.

Indurated papular primary sore of finger.

malignant disease, Behçet's syndrome and traumatic lesions. In addition, in the case of a tonsillar chancre, pyogenic infection, diphtheria, Vincent's infection, lesions occurring in agranulocytosis or reticulosis, and carcinoma must be excluded.

DIAGNOSIS OF CHANCRE

It should be strongly suspected that a lesion is syphilitic when there is, (1) a history of a long incubation period; (2) painless genital lesion; (3) firm, non-tender palpable lymph node in the drainage area. The diagnosis of early syphilitic chancre should *always* be made by dark-ground microscopy, *i.e.* by the demonstration of the *T. pallidum*, live, in the field. In the majority of cases at this stage the serum tests for specific antibody are negative.

Collection of Specimens

The exudate from a surface lesion, or the aspirate from enlarged regional lymph glands, is examined by dark-ground method. For satisfactory examination the specimen should be clear and contain the minimum of red blood cells or debris. In the case of an open sore it is important to obtain serum from the deeper aspects close to the margin, where the spirochaetes are most abundant. The suspected lesion is thoroughly cleansed with spirit or normal saline and finally mopped dry. Steady pressure is exerted at the base of the sore and if the exudate is at first obviously bloodstained, it should be wiped away and the pressure maintained until an adequate, clear specimen is obtained. If this yields little or no serum, one should scarify the edge of the ulcer. The exudate may be collected by a long capillary tube or by curette.

In the case of healed sores, aspiration, after injection of saline into the selected area of the periphery, yields good specimens. The technique is closely similar to that of gland puncture which may be employed in cases of healed or inaccessible sores. The selected gland is fixed between the forefinger and thumb and the point of a hypodermic needle is introduced obliquely through the skin and subcutaneous tissue into the substance of the gland. Saline 0·2 ml. may be injected. The gland is gently massaged and after a few moments suction is made. The serum is then transferred to a slide, a coverslip placed over it and pressed down. It is important that slides, of a thickness not more than 1 mm., and No. 1 cover-glasses, should be used for dark-ground work. The examination is repeated daily if necessary for three-days.

If the specimen has to be sent to a laboratory for examination, a capillary tube should be used. One end is gently stroked over the exuding lesion until the tube is filled to an extent of about 25 mm. The serum is shaken down towards the centre of the tube and both ends are sealed in a flame. Live *T. pallidum* may be recognised in this specimen even after several days.

Should the sore be secondarily infected the examination may be repeated when the patient has been treated with sulphonamides, either a long-acting sulphonamide (*e.g.* sulphamethoxydiazine), 1·0 g. a day, or a mixture such as sulphatriad 0·5 g. four-hourly, for three or four days.

IDENTIFICATION OF T. PALLIDUM

There are three genera in the family *Treponemataceae*: *Treponema*, *Borrelia* and *Leptospira*.

Treponema pallidum of syphilis can usually be differentiated with relative ease from other spirochaetes which may be encountered in specimens from genital or buccal sores by attention to morphology and characteristics of movement. *T. pallidum* has a delicate regular spiral (or possibly wave-form), varying in length from 6 μ to 18 μ, usually 7–12 μ, with a breadth of approximately 0·2 μ–0·25 μ. The spirals are narrow, measuring about 1 μ from crest to crest, the depth being slightly greater. The ends are pointed; possession of flagella is now considered doubtful. Under dark-ground illumination the colour appears dead white: motility across the microscope field is slow despite possible vigorous movements of a screw-like rotation about the long axis, slight expansion and closure of the coils, and 'angling' or bending on the long axis to more than a right-angle without loss of spiral form (p. 3). *T. pallidum* is morphologically indistinguishable from *T. pertenue*, the causal organism of yaws, which is one of the non-syphilitic treponematoses (p. 178).

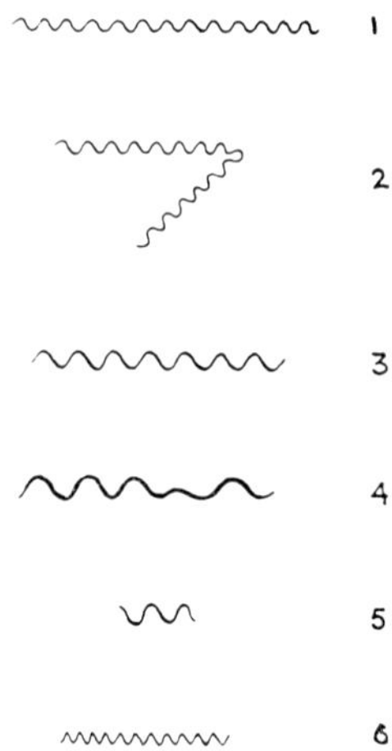

(1) *T. pallidum.*
(2) *T. pallidum* showing angling.
(3) *T. gracile.*
(4) *B. refringens.*
(5) *T. balanitidus.*
(6) *T. microdentium.*

Other treponemes which may be met with are: *T. balanitidis* (*genitalis*); *T. gracile*, coarser but very similar to *T. pallidum*; *T. microdentium*, smaller but very similar to *T. pallidum* without the screw-like motion or angling of the latter; *T. macrodentium*; *Borrelia buccalis*; *B. vincenti* appears together with fusiform bacilli when there are ulcerative buccal lesions; *T. refringens* occurs on the genitalia, appearing brighter, more active and coarser than other spirochaetes (see diagram above).

DARK-GROUND OIL IMMERSION MICROSCOPY

An ordinary bacteriological microscope, using $\frac{1}{12}$ in. oil objective, is modified by the inclusion of, (1) a funnel-stop or 'iris' in the oil immersion objective, and (2) a centre stop provided below the special Abbé condenser so that only peripheral rays are transmitted. Thus refractile objects in the microscopic field are illuminated against a black background. Special dark-ground condensers are available for this work.

To prepare the microscope for use, it is essential that the condenser be centred properly and that the funnel stop be in position in the objective lens. Immersion oil is applied to the surface of the condenser and to the upper surface of the coverslip of the preparation to be viewed. The condenser is brought up to the under surface of the slide and the objective lens down to the upper surface of the coverslip, there now being oil or fluid between all surfaces. Difficulties in focusing are frequently due to too great a thickness of slide or to inaccurate centring of the condenser.

CHAPTER 3

Early Infectious Syphilis (Secondary Syphilis) — Rash

From the moment that *T. pallidum* penetrates the skin or mucous membranes there is a steady progression towards generalisation of the infection. The organism extends at first by the lymphatics, and later enters the blood stream causing a true spirochaetaemia, in which every organ and tissue of the body is liable to invasion. Manifestations of this wide dissemination may occur within a few days of the appearance of the primary sore, or may be delayed for several months. The stage of syphilitic exanthem is characterised by constitutional symptoms and skin rashes. Infrequently, more serious involvement of the viscera occurs.

The constitutional symptoms, nearly always mild, and met with in about 25 per cent of patients, usually precede the onset of the skin rash. Diffuse headache, subject to nocturnal exacerbation, anorexia, nausea, constipation and bone, muscle or joint pains are the symptoms most frequently experienced. Fever of an intermittent or continuous type may occur: in these cases the temperature seldom rises above 37·8°–38·4° C. (100°–101° F.). Secondary anaemia and menstrual irregularities are frequent in women. Occasionally marked and more serious symptoms occur, such as persistent intense occipital headache, associated with stiffness of the neck, which may indicate early basal meningeal involvement. Transient albuminuria is not uncommon; acute nephritis is met with occasionally.

The eruption affecting the skin or mucous membranes is the most prominent feature of early generalised syphilis. While an almost infinite variety of clinical appearances may be met with, the early rashes fall into well-defined types and present definite characteristics. At first the roseole or macule is the individual element, while later it is the papule. The underlying pathology affords an explanation. When in the process of blood-stream dissemination, *T. pallidum* reaches the skin vessels, the same sequence of changes occurs as in the primary sore. The stage of

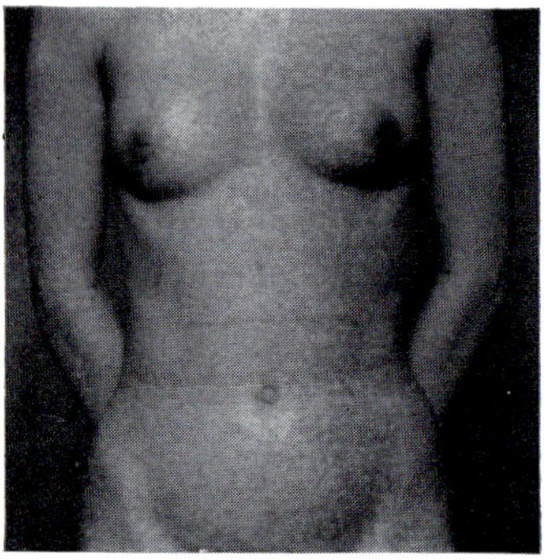

FIG. 31.
Early macular rash.

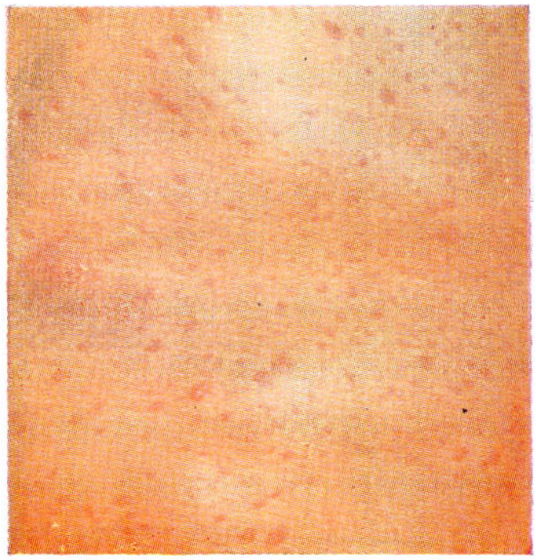

FIG. 32.
Maculo-papular rash.

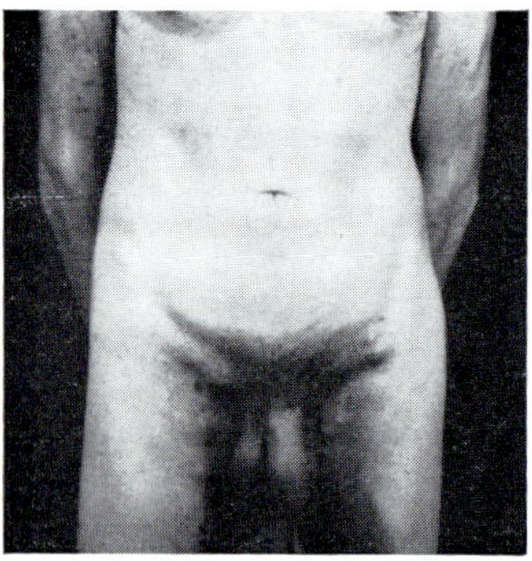

FIG. 33.
Maculo-papular rash, showing inguinal adenitis and oedema of prepuce over subpreputial chancre.

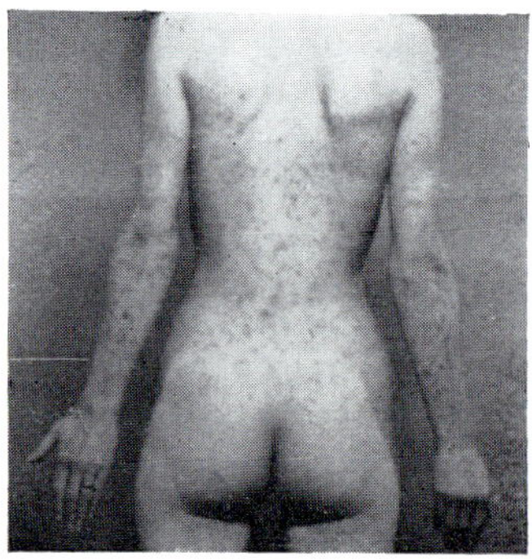

FIG. 34.
Papular rash.

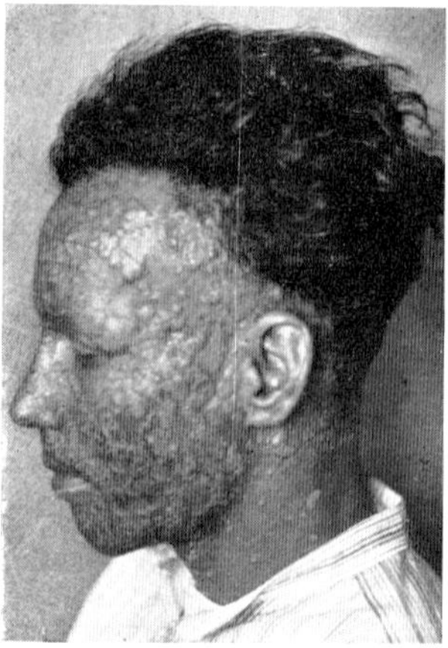

FIG. 35.
Smooth, non-scaly papular syphilide.

capillary dilatation with endothelial swelling and proliferation is recognisable clinically in the roseolar or macular rash (an allergic basis). The later perivascular cellular infiltration, partial or complete arterial occlusion, revascularisation and deposition of fibrous tissue gradually extending throughout the individual lesions, are manifested by the variations of the papular rash containing the treponeme.

DIAGNOSIS

The early roseola and the macular rash leave a symmetrical distribution affecting typically the flexor surfaces of the body. Macular rashes are commonly limited to chest, shoulders, flanks, abdomen and anus, and may be difficult to detect. Papular rashes involve in addition the face, palms and soles. The diameter of the early lesion is from 0·3 to 1·0 cm. As the lesions become papular their colour becomes dull copper or 'raw ham', later to become brownish red. In configuration the rash later tends to be patterned in circles or segments of circles. Papular lesions alone show induration (nodules), but are quite painless, and the rash as a whole does not irritate. Characteristic of syphilis is the *pleomorphism* of the rash—the occurrence at the same time, together, of different elements of skin rash.

Glandular enlargement is associated with the rash in almost all cases, and may even be noted in the absence of a generalised rash. The glands are not tender, but somewhat rubbery-firm in texture. The suboccipital, posterior cervical and epitrochlear groups are characteristically affected. Suppuration never occurs.

The *T. pallidum* is present in the papular eruption and in the lymph-nodes, and the specific serum tests are *always* positive at this stage.

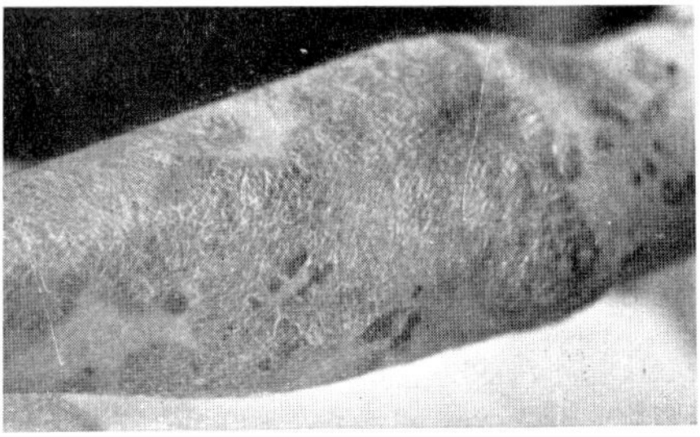

FIG. 36.

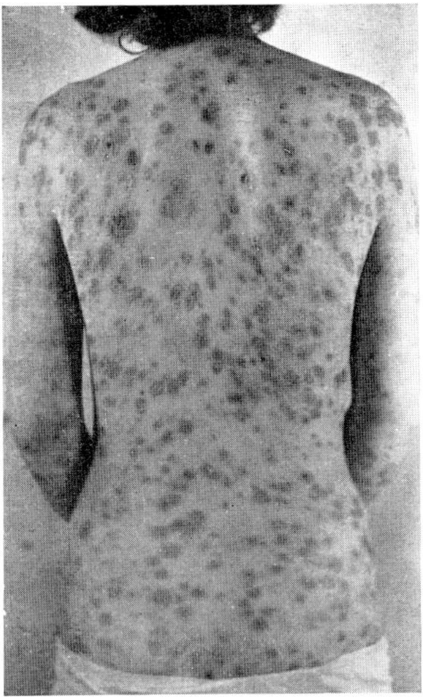

FIG. 37.

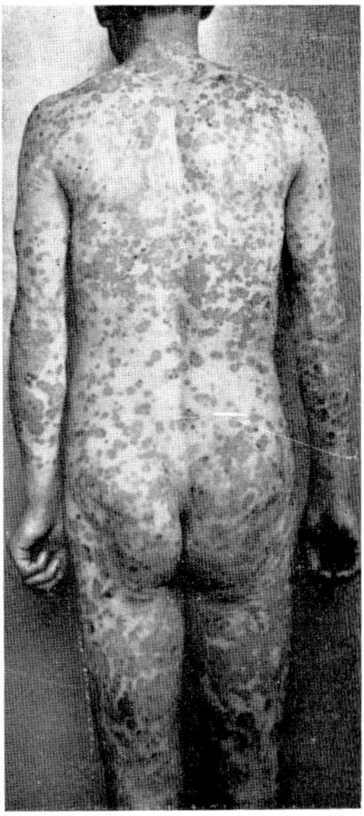

FIG. 38.

Diffuse papulo-squamous eruptions simulating psoriasis.

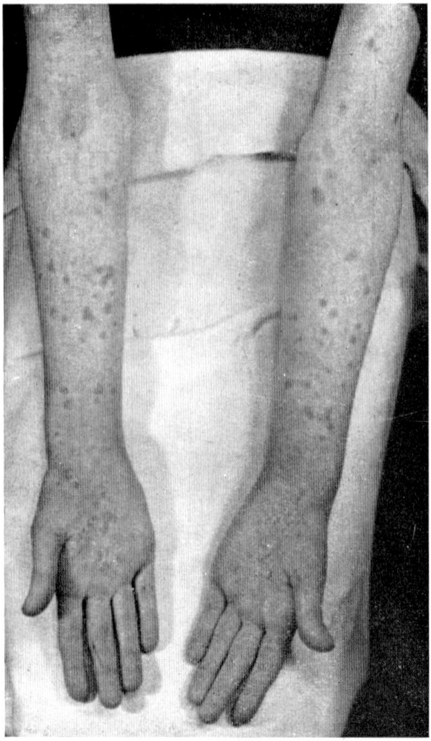

FIG. 39.

Papulo-squamous secondary rash of arms and palms.

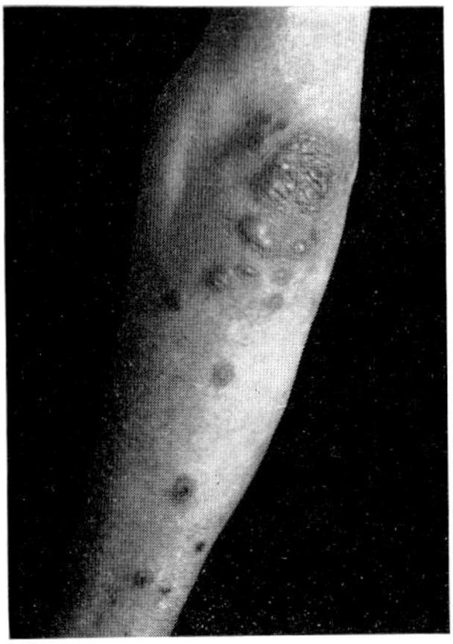

FIG. 40.

Pustular syphilide of the back of the elbow, showing unruptured and recently ruptured pustules.

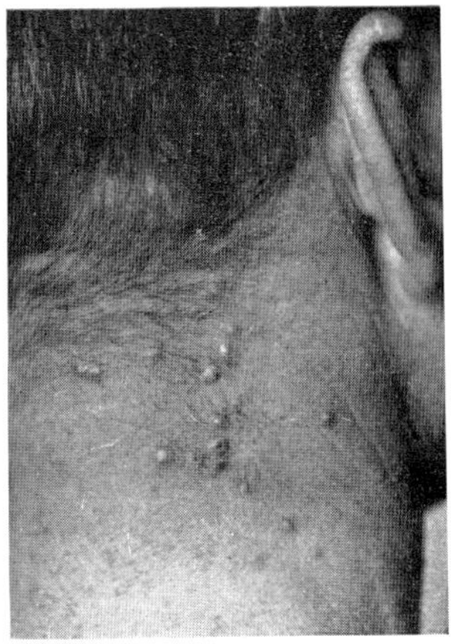

FIG. 41.

Pustular syphilide of neck where lesions suggest molluscum contagiosum.

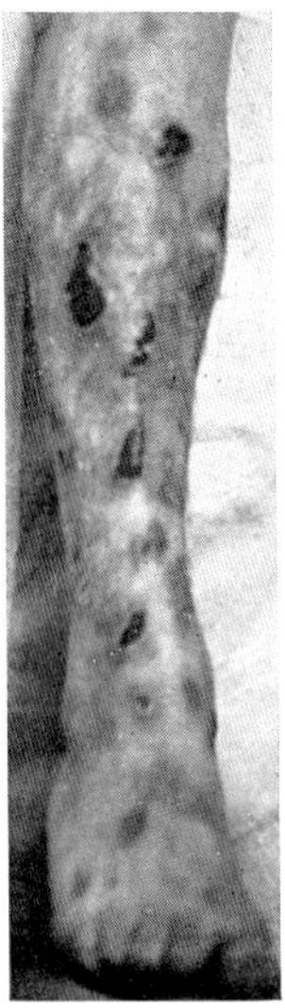

FIG. 42.

Widespread impetigenous syphilide of legs.

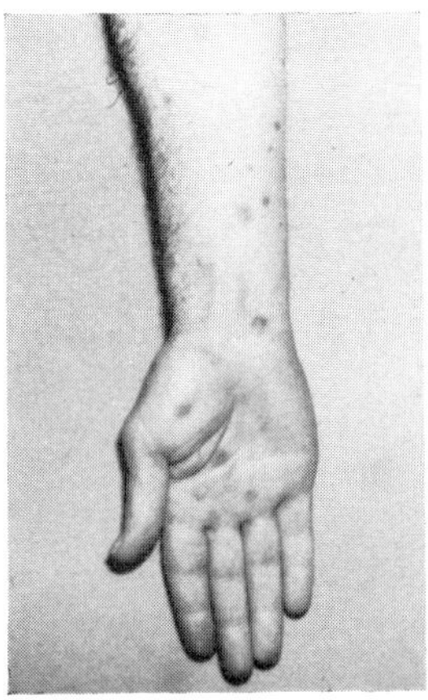

FIG. 43.

Palmar papules.

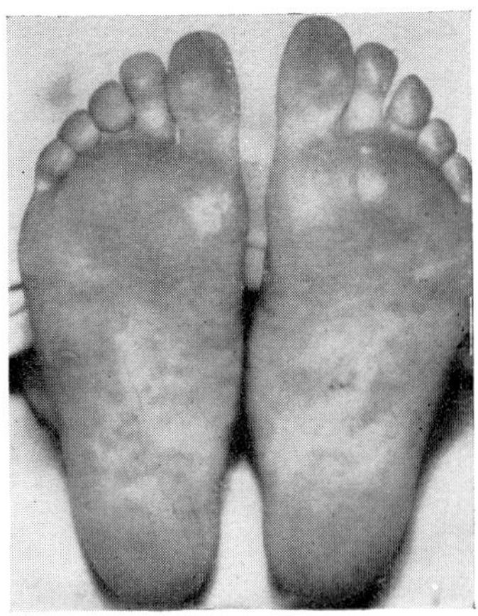

FIG. 44.

Plantar papules.

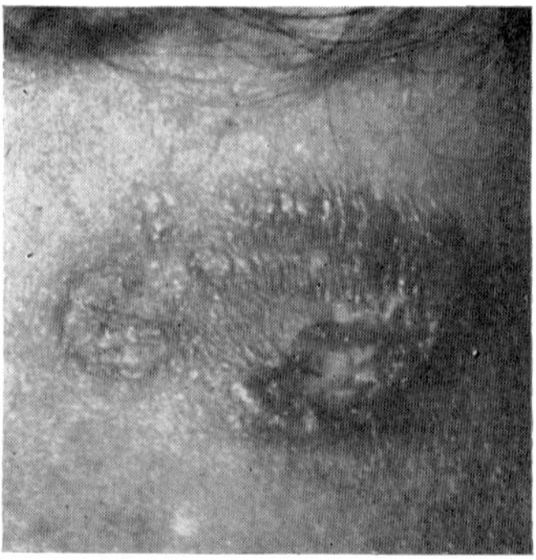

FIG. 45.

Crescentic syphilide of the neck, with early ulceration.

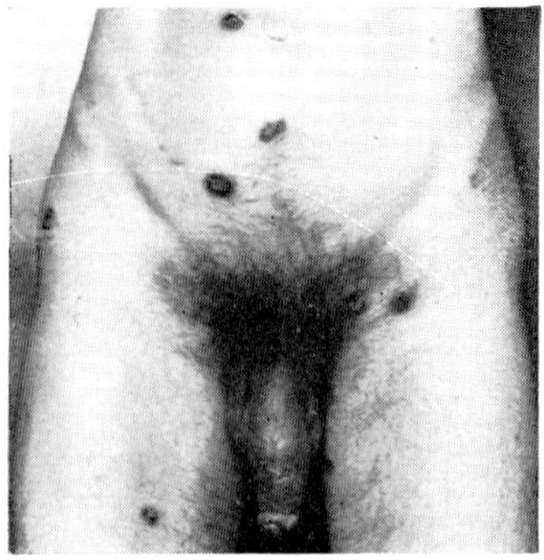

FIG. 46.

Ulcerative, ecthymatous secondary papular syphilide, occurring six months after infection.

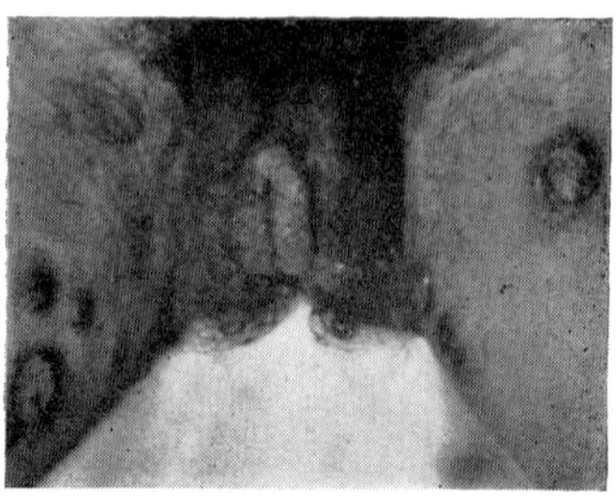

FIG. 47.

Rupial syphilide.

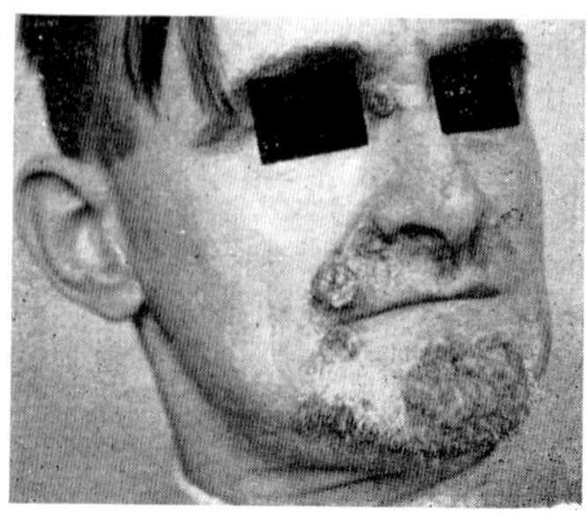

FIG. 48.

Hypertrophic syphilide. The lesions at the base of the nose shows granulomatous outgrowth.

DIFFERENTIAL DIAGNOSIS

1. The *roseolar rash* must be distinguished from the punctate bright red erythema of scarlet fever: a high pyrexia and a strawberry appearance to the tongue assists. In measles there are dull red, irregular and crescent macules coalescing into patches, together with pyrexia, coryza, conjunctivitis and Koplik's spots on the buccal mucosa. Rubella presents with posterior cervical and suboccipital lymphadenitis and a rose-coloured macular eruption fading in one to three days. Pityriasis rosea starts with a single oval 'herald patch', which is followed by the rash itself, consisting of red-pink macules, the lesions lying parallel to the long-axes of the ribs. Scaling is present. Glandular fever can present with a pink macular rash and enlarged lymph glands.

2. *Macular, maculo-papular and papular syphilides* occur as a further development of the early rash. There is a transition from the macular to the papular type of lesion. The macular syphilide is more or less pigmented, presenting either as, (*a*) pigmented macules, (*b*) diffuse hyperpigmentation with vitiligo or (*c*) loss of pigment in the macules: this leucoderma is pathognomonic of syphilis. Lesions are usually 0·3–1·0 cm. in diameter; they occur mainly in women and affect the region of the neck and shoulder. They are symptomless, indolent and pleomorphic. Small papular lesions affect the trunk, limbs and face, rarely the palms and soles. They are of a dull copper-red colour. Smooth papular syphilides may simulate lichen planus, which is violaceous in colour and neither indurated nor pleomorphic. The papular syphilide may be distributed in circles or segments of circles as an *annular syphilide*, which must be distinguished from granuloma annulare. Sometimes central ulceration leads to 'crusting' and impetigenous changes—*rupial syphilide*. More florid hypertrophic changes are uncommon: *framboesiform syphilide*.

Papular eczema presents as an irritable red, non-indurated, sometimes vesicular rash, typically affecting the extensor surfaces of the limbs, as does erythema multiforme. Drug rashes commonly occur on the trunk, neck and limbs, and result in various symptoms. They are often erythematous, urticarial or vesicular, and may be of pleomorphic type like erythema multiforme. Seborrhoeic dermatitis presents as irritable, yellowish, greasy, oval lesions, without infiltration, on chest, in the interscapular region and flexures. The scalp is affected. Psoriasis is distinguished by the red, scaly lesions particularly on the extensor aspects of the limbs. When the scale is removed multiple capillary bleeding points are found. Mainly nocturnal itching is typical of the lesions of scabies. The mite seeks the areas of the axillary folds, wrist creases and finger webs. Many cases are sexually transmitted, when the lesions may be limited to the lower abdomen, genitalia and thighs.

Mucous Membrane and Mucocutaneous Manifestations of Early Generalised Syphilis

At any time after the early generalisation of a syphilitic infection, and commonly with the appearance of the skin eruption, evidence may be found of involvement of the buccal mucous membrane or of the mucocutaneous junctions of the lips, nasal orifice, anus and vulva. These signs correspond to the maculopapular or papular skin eruption, modified by a moist area. Moist lesions are the most contagious of all syphilitic manifestations. Precaution must, therefore, be taken during the examination. The common manifestations are: a diffuse erythematous *pharyngitis*; *mucous patches*; moist papules in the mouth or throat; moist papules and *condylomata lata* in the anal and vulval regions. In most cases a diffuse erythematous pharyngitis occurs, and is frequently associated with tonsilitis and laryngitis. A 'chronic sore throat', with slight pain or discomfort and dysphagia, is complained of. The voice may be husky. Slight rise of temperature is found but the patient is less ill than would be expected. There are sometimes patches of thin, greyish exudate over the tonsils and pillars of the fauces. Enlargement of the posterior cervical and sub-occipital lymph glands is constant. Mucous patches or moist papules also occur.

Mucous patches correspond to the maculopapular early skin lesions. The lesions are circular in outline, varying in diameter

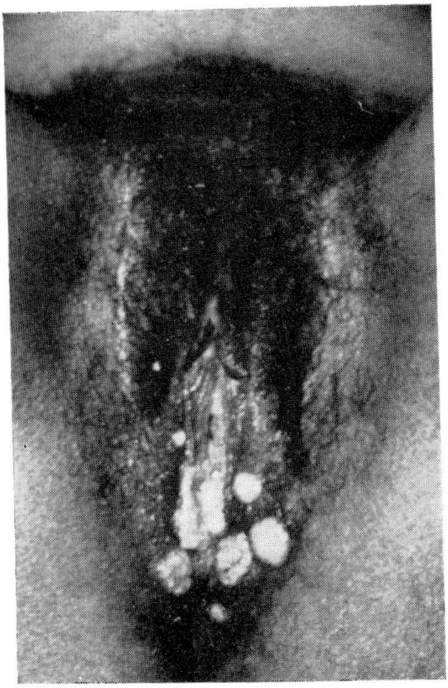

FIG. 49.
Vulval condylomata lata.

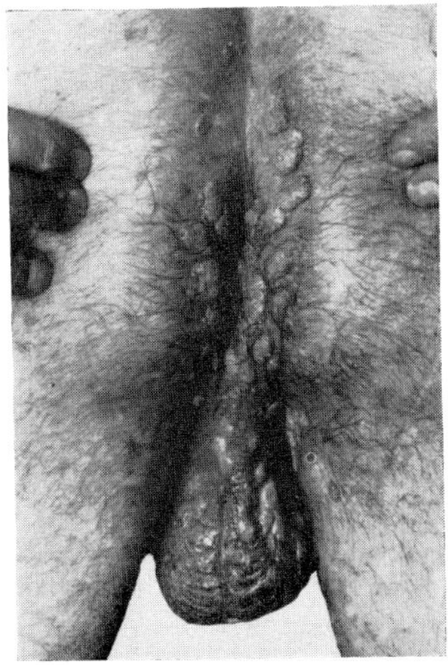

FIG. 50.
Condylomata lata of anus, inner aspect of buttocks, and scrotum.

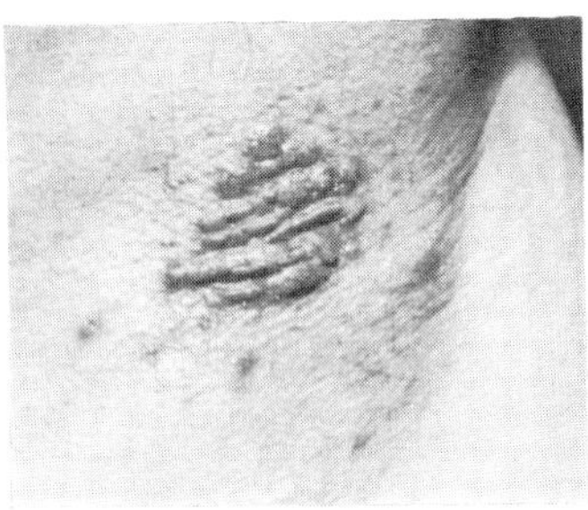

FIG. 51.
Moist papules in axilla.

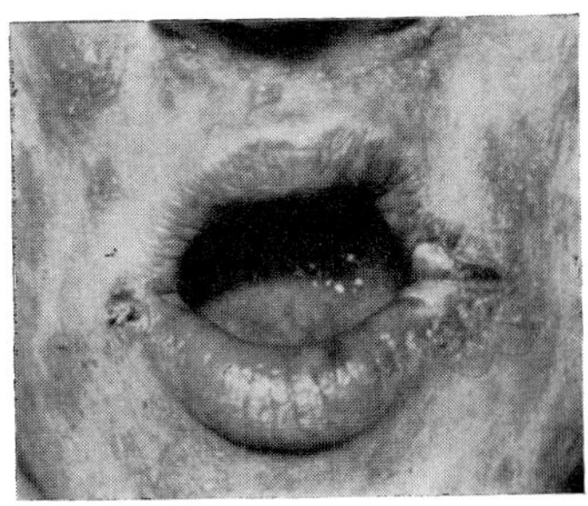

FIG 52.
Syphilitic angular stomatitis.

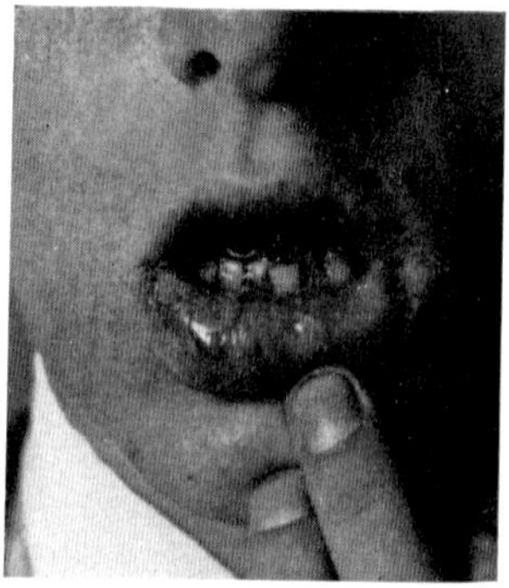

FIG. 53.

Mucous patches of inner aspect of lower lip with commencing peripheral erosion.

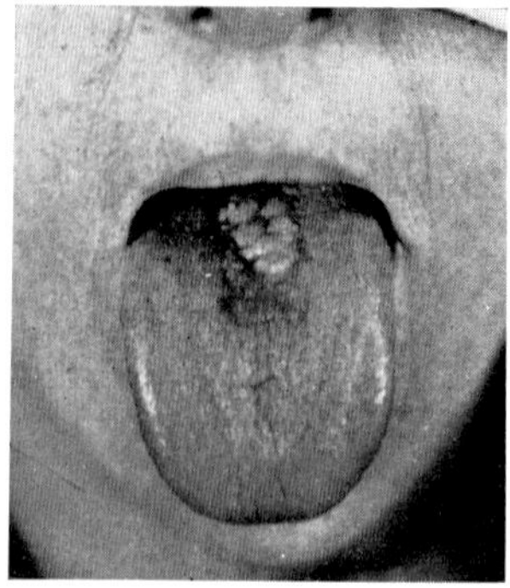

FIG. 54.

Moist papules of dorsum of tongue.

up to 1 cm., and have slightly raised milky or greyish flat tops. There is no induration of the base. Erosion of the surface occurs rapidly, with, at first, a peripheral red rim. Ulceration seldom takes place except as the result of irritation from carious teeth or from pyogenic infection. The common sites, in order of frequency, are the inner aspect of the lips, especially at the angles, the tonsils, the gums, the dorsum and under-surface of the tongue, the hard and soft palate.

Moist patches in the mouth have a similar distribution. Central necrosis is frequent, causing ulcers with a slightly raised edge and dull red base. Coalescence of mucous patches or moist papules in circinate or serpiginous formation frequently occurs on the tonsils, giving rise to typical '*snail-track*' *ulcers*. At the nasal and oral mucocutaneous junctions moist papules generally remain discrete, but tend to become hypertrophic and often develop a wart-like appearance.

Condylomata lata represent further hypertrophic development of the moist papule. In the peri-anal area and on the inner aspect of the labia majora they become flat-topped, raised, broad-based lesions of a greyish-white colour. In patients of uncleanly habits they may extend to the perineum and scrotum in the male, and to the perineum, natal cleft and inner aspect of the thighs in the female. Coalescence may give rise to sessile vegetative plaques.

Moist papules or condylomata lata may occur on the potentially moist areas of the skin, *e.g.* in the axilla, underneath the pendulous female breast and in the web of the fingers or toes. They may present as the only external manifestation of early infectious syphilis.

DIFFERENTIAL DIAGNOSIS

The 'sore throat' of early syphilis must be distinguished from acute tonsilitis or, if there is much obvious membrane formation, from diphtheria and Vincent's angina. The chronic course and mild constitutional symptoms should suggest the possibility of syphilis. The serum tests are always positive.

Mucous patches and moist papules have to be differentiated, before erosion, from thrush, the mucosal lesions of certain skin diseases, *e.g.* lichen planus, and from the buccal lesions accompanying skin rashes. After erosion differentiation must be made from aphthous ulcers, herpes simplex and the buccal manifestations of erythema multiforme. Condylomata lata have to be distinguished from condylomata acuminata (or virus warts) and from pemphigus vegetans. Condylomata acuminata may be sessile or pedunculated, but there is no induration of the base, the surface is frequently cauliflower-like and lacks the moist greyish top of condylomata lata.

The diagnosis of the mucocutaneous lesions in secondary syphilis depends upon the clinical recognition with evidence of syphilis affecting the skin, genitalia or lymphatic glands, the demonstration of *T. pallidum* and the presence of positive *serological tests* for syphilis.

Affections of the Hair

Changes affecting the nails may occur during the early generalised stage and also in late syphilis. Together with the maculopapular or papular skin rash similar eruptions occur on the scalp, giving rise to papular, pustular, impetigenous or even rupial

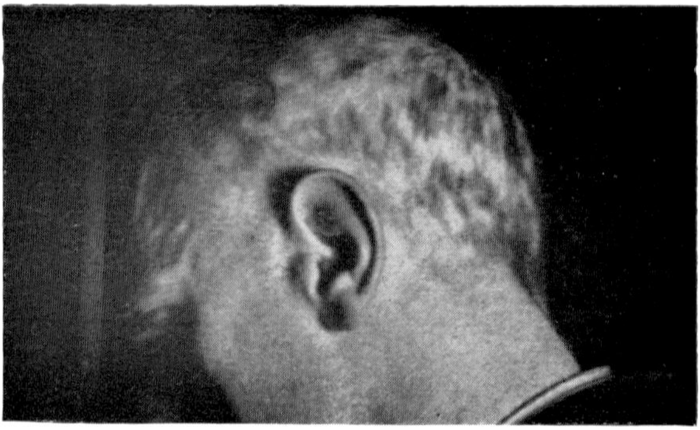

FIG. 55—Syphilitic alopoecia; typical 'moth-eaten' appearance.

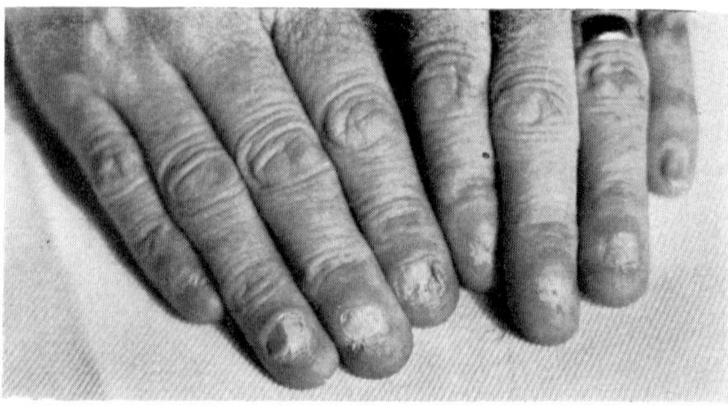

FIG. 56. Syphilitic onychia.

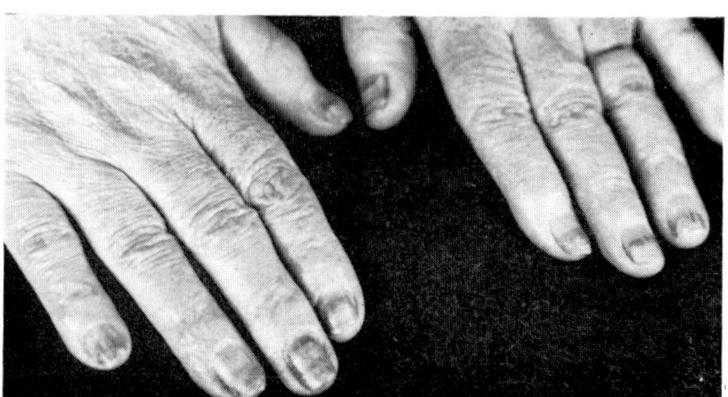

FIG. 57. Syphilitic onychia.

lesions. There may be a generalised thinning of the hair, or syphilitic alopecia, which is most marked on the back and sides of the head and gives rise to a patchy, 'moth-eaten' appearance. The ill-defined distribution of the loss of hair and the absence of 'exclamation mark' hairs should avoid any confusion with alopecia areata. Usually complete recovery is made under systemic treatment: occasionally, however, a permanent baldness results.

Affections of the Nails

Nail lesions may occur during the secondary period, but are more common in late syphilis: (1) a brittle condition of the nail develops and the free border becomes notched or serrated. In some cases the brittleness is associated with hypertrophic thickening. (2) There may be pitting of the dorsal surface, the pits commencing as small, whitish areas on the dorsum of the nail which, when removed, leave blackened, rough depressions in the nail plate. (3) Symptomless exfoliation of the entire nail may occur. (4) Papular or pustular lesions of the nail bed: the colour gradually changes to yellow, the overlying nail becomes thin and crumbles away leaving a gap. Often only one nail is involved. (5) Paronychia begins as a redness and swelling round the nail bed, pain being less marked than in pyogenic infection. Syphilitic paronychia commonly results in permanent deformity of the affected nails or, infrequently, in their complete loss. (6) In late generalised syphilis symmetrically distributed spoon-shaped nails are occasionally seen and are pathognomonic.

Visceral Involvement

Constitutional symptoms are found in less than half the cases in the generalised stage, and are almost always mild. A few of these, however, are accompanied by syphilitic lesions in the various viscera. Apart from the skin and the lymphatic system, which are so frequently involved, signs in other systems may also occur: *Osseous*: localised tender spots may be present, most commonly in the tibia, due to periostitis. *Viscera*: nephritis; albuminuria, and occasionally casts may be noted in the urine, the renal function showing little impairment. Rarely, small nodules may form in the *epididymis* at this stage. Enlargement of the liver, with or without mild icterus, is infrequently met with; splenic enlargement however is less rare. *Central nervous system*: the nervous system is often involved in the absence of signs or symptoms and about a third of cases of early generalised syphilis have an abnormal C.S.F. The number increases to over 50 per cent in the 'late secondary' stage. The signs of *early neurosyphilitic* involvement are irritative, due to meningitis. There may also be loss of function because of spread of inflammation from the meninges, with involvement of the cranial nerves or, more rarey, of the brain or spinal cord. *Cardiovascular*: although involvement of the cardia is thought to occur during the early stages of syphilis there is no satisfactory proof for it.

Lesions of the *eye* may be noted and include conjunctivitis, iritis, non-granulomatous or granulomatous, and, rarely, optic neuritis. Involvement of the *ear* is also rare in the early stages of syphilis.

Early Latent Syphilis

An unknown number of infected persons harbour the organism without any clinical signs of their infection developing in the early stages. They therefore are a danger to themselves, being liable to suffer from any of the lesions of late syphilis, and are a possible danger to their sexual partners. A 'latent' period also occurs in the natural history of the disease after the clearing of the signs of early general rash, which takes place in many untreated patients in a matter of two to six months.

Duration of Infectiousness of Untreated Early Syphilis

The disease is infectious when early lesions are present. During the stage of generalised rash most of the body secretions carry such a risk. Infectiousness declines during the first year and in most cases becomes negligible in the course of the second year. But women may infect a foetus many years after they themselves became infected. Infected blood donors also carry a risk.

Treatment

The treatment of early infectious syphilis should render the lesions non-contagious in one to two days, thus removing the risk to others, and should effect a complete eradication of the infection in the individual. This is done by giving the patient sufficient treatment, and proving its adequacy by regular observation of the patient over the following two years. There is evidence that minimal, inadequate treatment in the early stages predisposes to later visceral manifestations.

Management of the case is important. The aim is to cure the disease in every case. The general health of the patient ought to be maintained throughout treatment and observation. Local treatment is simple and confined to general cleansing using normal saline, 1/8000 potassium permanganate, simple dusting powder or lotions such as calamine.

Specific treatment for early syphilis today is extremely effective. Antibiotics are used and pencillin by injection is still the most widely exhibited and successful of these drugs. It is best given by intramuscular injection. It can be used in aqueous solution (as benzylpenicillin G) every four hours or, better, given in the form of one of the repository penicillins, which are slowly released from the depôt in the muscles. The total dosage for early infectious syphilis should be approximately 10 million units by intramuscular injection; raised to 14 million units in the more severe cases or heavy and large patients.

A recommended treatment for the average case is the use of the procaine salt of penicillin G: 900,000 units (in phials, 300,000 units per ml.) of this preparation are injected intramuscularly daily for 10 days. An alternative method is to use one of the longer-acting penicillin preparations (such as benzathine penicillin) which need only be administered in the requisite dosage every four days or at longer intervals. The course is repeated if necessary (p. 43) and it has to be borne in mind that, although most patients respond well and rapidly to therapy, occasionally this does not happen, sometimes with disastrous results. Oral penicillin is unsatisfactory for the treatment of syphilis.

An acute hypersensitivity reaction, following the release of treponemal antigen into the system soon after the start of treatment, and known as the *Jarisch-Herxheimer* reaction, occurs in half of all cases of early syphilis, especially in those who have a syphilitic rash. It is a febrile reaction, accompanied by malaise, headache and an exacerbation of signs, irrespective of the dose of penicillin employed. It is of no serious consequence in early syphilis, but can result in serious damaging effects in late syphilis.

If the patient is sensitised to penicillin, *tetracycline* is available. For early syphilis tetracycline is taken by mouth, 2·0 g. daily, 0·5 g. every six hours, not within an hour of a meal in order to obtain maximum absorption, for a total of 14 days. Careful clinical and serological observation should be made of its effects on the disease. Tetracycline being an antibiotic with so wide a range of usefulness, it must be remembered that, in children, it can result in pigmentation and hypoplasia of dental enamel, malformation of cusps and dental caries; it is also retained in the long bones, resulting in inhibition of linear growth. Teratogenic activity is doubtful; nevertheless the drug should be used with restraint in pregnancy.

Erythromycin may also be given, 3·0 g. daily dosage, but its effectiveness is less certain than that of tetracycline. Cephaloridine is a more successful alternative drug to penicillin in the treatment of syphilis, and is used in a dose of 2·0 g. every 24 hours, by intramuscular injection, for a total of 10 days.

Intramuscular Injection

All patients should be asked whether they have received penicillin before and if they have suffered from an allergy of any kind. The site generally chosen for intramuscular injection is the *upper and outer* gluteal quadrant. The technique of intramuscular injection is well known (p. 195).

Should the patient have an acute anaphylactic reaction to the injection, he or she should at once be laid flat, with head low. Treatment for severe reactions of this kind (syncopal) may require an injection of 1 : 1000 liq. adrenaline hydrochloride

(0·5 ml. subcutaneously or intramuscularly), or antihistamine drug (*e.g.* chlorpheniramine maleate 10 mg./ml. intramuscularly), or hydrocortisone (25–100 mg./ml. intramuscularly), to be repeated or given intravenously if necessary. In emergency such drugs should be given by the intravenous route.

OBSERVATION AFTER TREATMENT

After treatment the patient enters upon a period of surveillance of at least two years. Clinical and serological examinations should be repeated at first at intervals of one to three months, later less frequently. Great attention should be paid to the central nervous system and the cardiovascular system. Before the patient is discharged, clinical examination must be supplemented by examination of the *cerebrospinal fluid* if there is a doubt about the clinical or serological response of the patient.

The serological response, especially if gauged by a quantitative Wassermann or other 'standard' test, affords a valuable guide to the effectiveness of the antibiotic therapy. A decision to re-treat largely depends upon whether a satisfactory fall in serological titre has or has not taken place. The behaviour of the post-treatment serological tests falls into a number of typical patterns:—

SEROLOGICAL RESPONSE TO TREATMENT USING 'STANDARD TESTS'

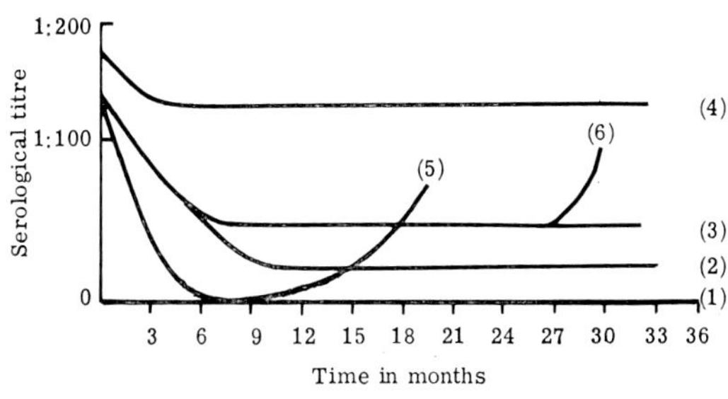

Graph showing:—

1. Serological negativity at fourteenth week.
2. Negativity delayed until the twelfth month.
3. Persistent low-positive serological titre.

4. Persistent high-positive serological titre.
5. Sero-relapse, usually within 12 months of treatment.
6. Sero-reactivation of a persistent positive test.

Sero-relapse and sero-reactivation are, of course, clear indications for *retreatment*. Retreatment however, with much larger doses, should also be considered whenever there are clinical or serological responses to treatment which are unduly slow or incomplete.

PROPHYLAXIS

Syphilis is satisfactorily treated by comparatively small doses of antibiotic during the incubation period of the disease. When a patient has run the risk of infection and desires treatment, of a prophylactic nature, it is thus tempting to administer such a drug. On the whole, however, this should be resisted, since, if such treatment is resorted to, the patient has to remain under observation for the usual period of two years, just as if the diagnosis had first been made.

An early potential case should receive 2·4 mega-units (8 ml.) procaine penicillin in one or two intramuscular injections. Benzathine penicillin may be used in its place. In the later weeks of the incubation period the dose should be 6·0 mega-units.

In a few localities the risk of contracting syphilis is unusually high. It is best therefore to examine the patient's serum at six and 12 weeks in order to exclude the disease, and only treat *after* diagnosis.

SERUM TESTS FOR SYPHILIS

These are tests for syphilitic antibody made on the patient's serum. Antibodies against antigens present in the *T. pallidum* appear in the serum of some patients from the third or fourth week of infection onwards. Antibodies are always present in cases of syphilis when the general rash appears. Thus in about one-third of well developed syphilitic chancres the serum tests will be negative. In late syphilis there is a similar tendency to find negative serum tests in some cases, especially, that is, with tests of the standard type.

Two types of serum test exist, the 'standard' tests, using non-specific lipo-protein as antigen, which detect 'pseudo-antibody', and the specific tests, using treponemal antigen.

The standard tests are still performed as a routine. These usually consist of the Wassermann reaction (W.R.) which is a complement fixation reaction; and either a Price's precipitation (PPR) or a Kahn or a VDRL reaction. The techniques of these tests are described on p. 204. Though reliable the standard tests are not absolutely specific and, occasionally, are positive in other conditions. Of the two types of standard test the W.R. is generally less sensitive than either the PPR or the Kahn reaction. These standard tests may be positive a little sooner in early infectious syphilis than the specific tests, and they tend to respond earlier to treatment.

The specific tests in use today are the Reiter protein complement fixation test (RPCFT), a technique similar to that of the W.R. but using a *treponemal* antigen; the Treponemal immobilisation test (TPI), in which live organisms are used; and the Fluorescent treponemal antibody test (FTA). The first of these is in almost routine use, the lyophilised antigen being supplied commercially. These tests are specific for all treponemal diseases, hence they do not distinguish one from another (*e.g.* syphilis from yaws). Although not all three tests will be found to be positive in every case, the area of disagreement in practice is very small indeed.

The group of patients in whom a positive W.R. occurs in the absence of syphilis, that is, in the absence of positive RPCFT, TPI and FTA tests, are termed *non-syphilitic reactors*. This type of result occurs, (1) as an acute or temporary phenomenon after inoculations, in allergy, following virus and rickettsial infection, mononucleosis, etc.; (2) in certain chronic or relapsing infections such as leprosy and malaria, and chronic disease of the liver; and (3) less commonly in certain of the so-called collagen disorders, especially disseminated lupus erythematosus. A positive W.R. therefore is usually due to syphilis, and in any case is always a reflection of a disorder in which there is some alteration in the serum proteins.

The results of serum tests run parallel to the clinical manifestations of syphilis. Furthermore they enable a diagnosis of *latent syphilis* to be made. When the patient proceeds beyond the stage of early generalisation of the infection, and either spontaneously recovers, in a few cases, or passes into a phase of latent syphilis, or alternatively develops visceral destructive lesions, the serum tests usually reflect the change.

In early generalised syphilis *all* the tests are strongly positive, both the 'standard' and the 'specific' tests. As time goes by and the character of the disease alters, so does the reactivity of the patient's serum change. The overall pattern of positivity may be conflicting or may vary, not only within the groups of tests themselves but over periods of time.

If there is any great degree of *activity* in late syphilis these tests will always reflect it; such as for example in cardiovascular syphilis, or parenchymatous neurosyphilis. But in certain situations of minimal infection or tissue activity the results of the serological tests may be equivocal or show variable patterns. It is considered probable that persistence of any quantity of antibody reflects the presence of live *T. pallidum* somewhere in the body; although the organism may be 'contained' by the body defences and by treatment, and the syphilis itself be inactive or quiescent. Moderately high positive titres are an indication for re-appraisal of the case, and if necessary retreatment with larger doses of antibiotic for three weeks, preceded by prednisolone (unless contraindicated) 45 mg. daily for a week which is 'tailed off' (p. 164) when the antibiotic is started.

Some well-treated cases of late syphilis, however, will retain their strong positive serological titres for many years, possibly for life. It is as well to administer to such patients relatively large amounts of antibiotic.

The serum tests are not uncommonly negative in the presence of active progressive syphilis when the two types of test are being performed: this was more likely to happen when, before the specific tests were evolved, only the standard tests were performed. Yet, in recent years, as has been pointed out, treponemes have been isolated in cases of treated late syphilis even when the serological tests have been negative.

Syphilitic antibody is transferred to the foetus through the placental capillaries. The infant thus possesses maternal antibody and pseudo-antibody persisting for four or more weeks after birth. Specific serum tests will therefore only reflect the presence of disease in the *infant* if performed on the infant six weeks or later following birth.

Pregnancy itself is probably not a direct cause of a positive W.R. in a women, despite the fact that serum lipid changes occur during this period. A positive 'standard' test in pregnancy is due either to a treponemal infection or to one of the known causes of a non-syphilitic reaction.

COLLECTION OF BLOOD

In adults blood is most conveniently obtained by vein puncture (p. 192).

In very young children blood may be obtained from a scalp or the anterior jugular vein. Alternatively, blood may be obtained by 'heel-stab' (p. 193).

CHAPTER 4

Late Syphilis (Tertiary Syphilis)

INTRODUCTION

In the absence of diagnosis and treatment, the manifestations of early generalised syphilis run their course in three to nine months and usually disappear spontaneously. The defensive mechanism of the body has, for the most part, eliminated the treponeme from the blood stream and from many of the tissues or organs of the body. Complete eradication of the parasite is, however, not accomplished in more than a small proportion of cases; a state of equilibrium is reached between the tissues and the infecting organism, and the spirochaete is confined to a number of residual foci, by the cellular immunity that develops.

During this phase of the disease, which follows early asymptomatic syphilis as well as symptomatic syphilis, there is produced both humoral antibody, reflected by the presence of positive serological tests, and a tissue sensitivity to the treponeme. Tissue *hyper*sensitivity not infrequently develops, and the lesions which occur are typified by that of the syphilitic gumma.

The attainment of a stage of equilibrium leads to an 'asymptomatic' period, when it follows early generalised syphilis, or perpetuates such a state when it follows early asymptomatic syphilis. It may vary in length from a few months up to 50 years or more: the condition is known as *latent syphilis*.

So long as residual foci of treponemes persist in the body, together with an altered tissue reactivity, there may be, (1) slowly progressive damage to the tissue involved (*e.g.* aorta, liver, central nervous system), and (2) recurrent episodes of spirochaetaemia.

The late manifestations of syphilis may conveniently be considered according to the systems involved under the following headings:—

1. Skin, mucosa, bone, joint, muscle lesions.
2. Cardiovascular and visceral lesions.
3. Neurosyphilis.
4. 'Asymptomatic' infection—Late latent syphilis.

While lesions affecting a number of tissues or organs may appear simultaneously, it is more usual to find only one system involved. In view, however, of the gravity of cardiovascular syphilis and neurosyphilis it is of the utmost importance to make routine, clinical and special investigations of these systems in every case of late syphilis coming under observation.

HISTOPATHOLOGY

The essential lesion of late (tertiary) syphilis is the formation of syphilitic granulation tissue. There is a balance in the progressive disease between the hyperimmune (gumma) cellular type of response and the more plastic or fibrotic response, one or the other seeming to predominate. Cellular infiltration with lymphocytes and plasma cells takes place in relation to lymphatics accompanying small blood vessels. There is a specific periarteritis, leading to endarteritis, resulting in reduced blood supply and tissue necrosis. Whereas there is a tendency for all early syphilitic lesions to resolve, this is not the case in late syphilis. These tissue changes are often of the cellular type, or what is known as the *gummatous* reaction, and form the basis of many late syphilitic lesions.

Mucocutaneous Manifestations

Mucous patches, moist papules, and condylomata lata may be met with in an *early recurrence*. The later the manifestations appear the greater is the tendency to asymmetrical distribution and to solitary lesions, or lesions localised to one area of the body. The mucocutaneous manifestations of *late* syphilis may be classified as:—

1. Nodular—non-ulcerative
   —ulcerative
2. Squamous
3. Gummatous (gummous)

Cutaneous Lesions

Nodular cutaneous syphilides begin as lesions in the corium increasing slowly in size (usually 0·5–2 cm. diameter), taking from one to three months to develop. The sites commonly affected are the nose, forehead, chin, neck, back, buttocks, and outer aspects of the thighs.

The lesions are circular in outline, and may be solitary or grouped, or present as typical serpiginous patches. They can be palpated as firm, elastic, sharply circumscribed nodules involving the entire thickness of the skin. The surface is of a reddish-brown or coppery colour, and is usually smooth and non-scaly. Fine desquamation can appear. The nodules may remain localised and persist without apparent change for a year or more. Commonly central necrosis and peripheral spread occurs, resulting in either deep, circular, 'punched-out' ulcers with sharp edges and a base covered with crusts or exudate, or healing with non-contractile atrophic scar tissue; there may be a spread of the solitary and grouped nodular lesions. The area of skin over which the spread has taken place may be apparently unaltered or may show atrophic, squamous, cicatricial, crustaceous or ulcerative changes. Alteration of pigmentation, (increase or decrease) is not infrequent in those cases in which otherwise apparently normal skin is left.

The larger the nodules and the more closely they are set together, the greater the possibility of ulceration and subsequent scar tissue formation. While the rate of spread is slow, wide areas of skin may be involved before the patient seeks advice. The process is usually unattended by any general upset.

DIAGNOSIS

Nodular cutaneous syphilides have to be differentiated from other conditions giving rise to nodular or raised lesions on the skin, *e.g.* urticaria, eczema, tuberculosis, sebaceous cysts, lipomata, fibromata, granuloma annulare. The spreading circinate or serpiginous lesions have to be distinguished from seborrhoea, psoriasis, ringworm, rosacea, lupus erythematosus, lupus vulgaris, mycosis fungoides, leprosy and epithelioma. The

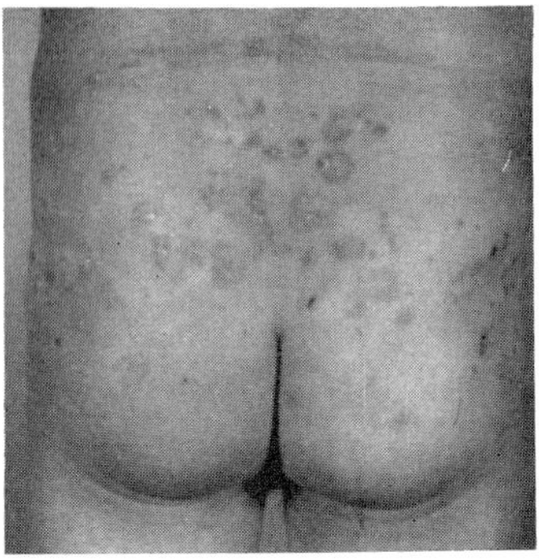

FIG. 58.

Annular syphilide showing crescentic figures.

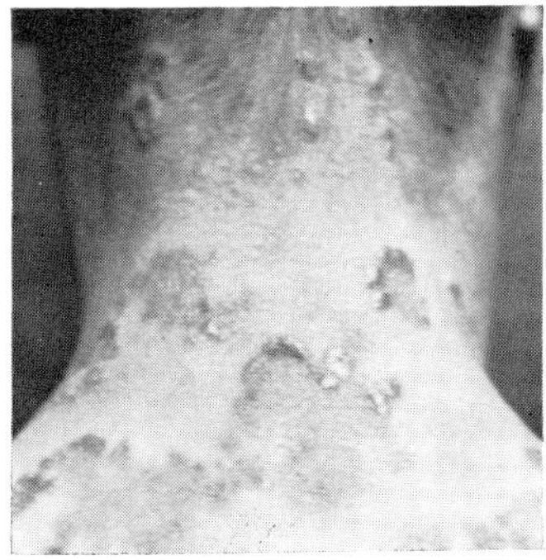

FIG. 59.

Nodular cutaneous syphilide two years after infection.

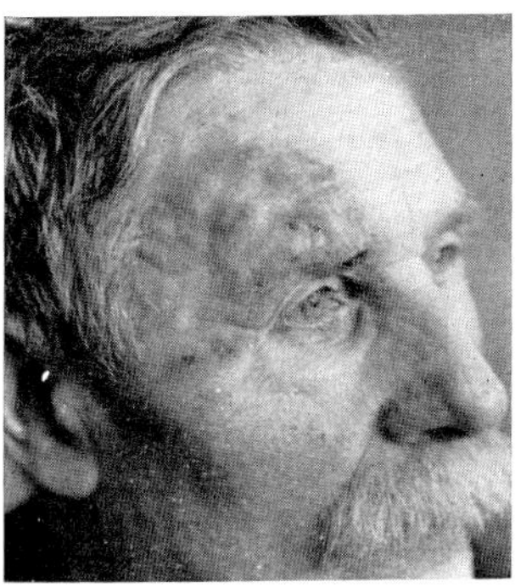

FIG. 60.

Nodular cutaneous syphilide of the temple following blow some three months previously.

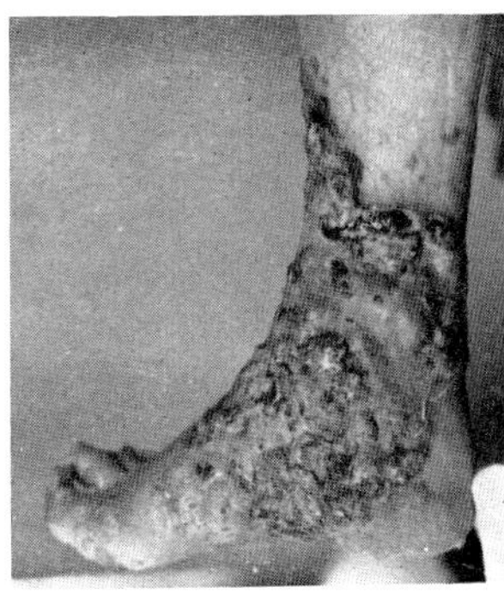

FIG. 61.

Nodular cutaneous eruption involving foot and ankle, duration five years; showing proliferation with many areas of ulceration.

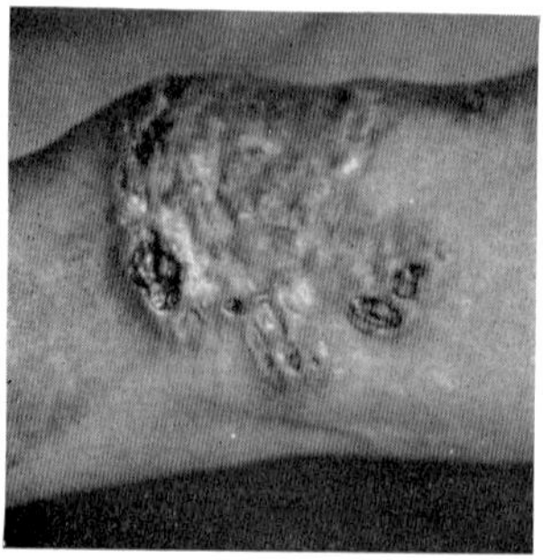

FIG. 62.

Ulcerative nodular cutaneous syphilide of knee.

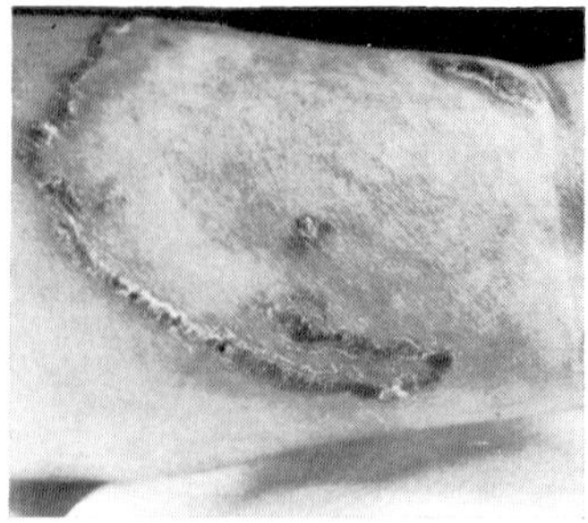

FIG. 63.

Gyrate (serpiginous) late syphilis.

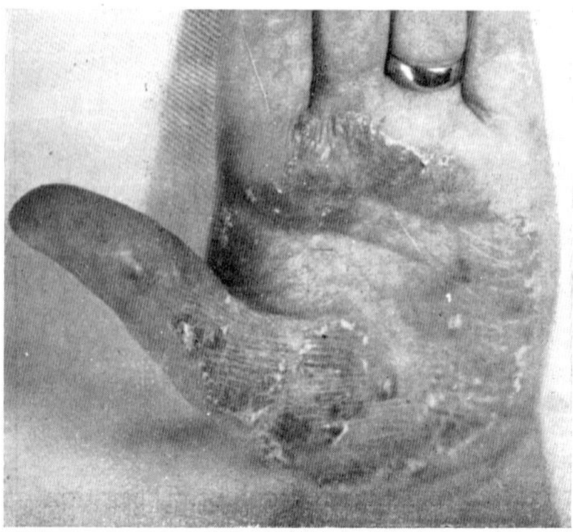

FIG. 64.

Squamous syphilides are nodular cutaneous syphilides affecting the palms or soles.

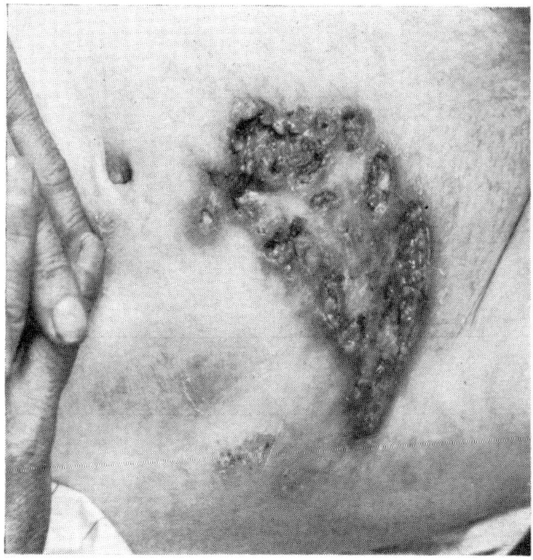

FIG. 65.

Nodular cutaneous syphilide of right hypogastrium; ulcerative phase predominant.

asymptomatic, slowly progressive, sharply defined, indurated nodular lesions of late syphilis, occurring in circles or segments of circles, the 'punched-out' ulceration, and atrophic non-contractile scars, should suggest the possible diagnosis.

Squamous syphilides (palmar or plantar syphilides)

The occurrence of nodular cutaneous syphilides on the palms or soles gives rise to well-defined, diffuse or localised scaling lesions of circular outline and dull red colour. Ulceration or fissuring never occurs. The squamous syphilides have to be *differentiated* from the manifestations of eczema, psoriasis, and ringworm.

CUTANEOUS GUMMA

While the nodular cutaneous syphilides are intracutaneous gummata, the true gumma commences as a small, firm, painless, circumscribed nodule in the subcutaneous or deeper structures,

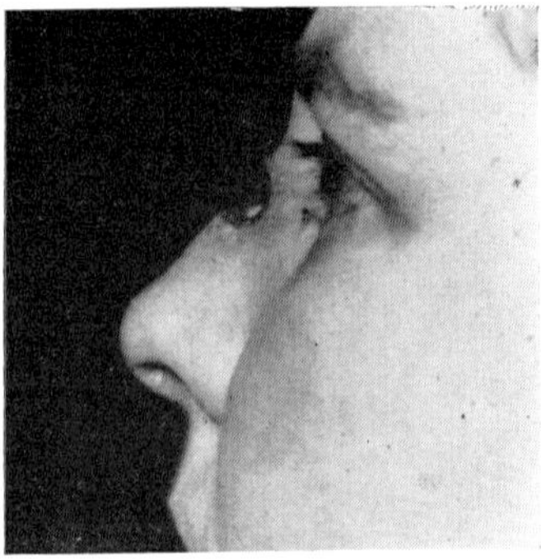

FIG. 66.

Early gummatous ulceration of the bridge of the nose.

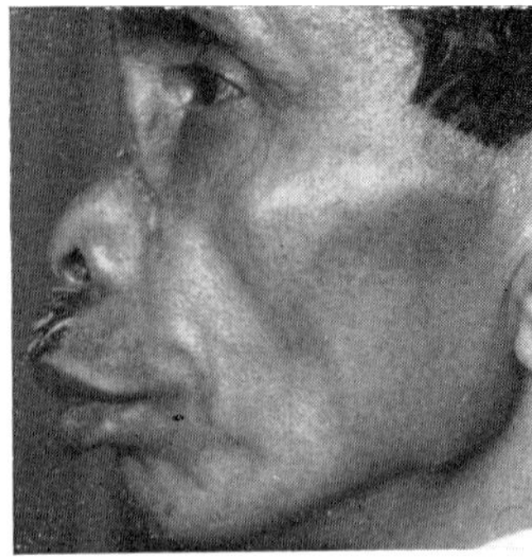

FIG. 67.

Results of gummatous destruction of the nasal bridge.

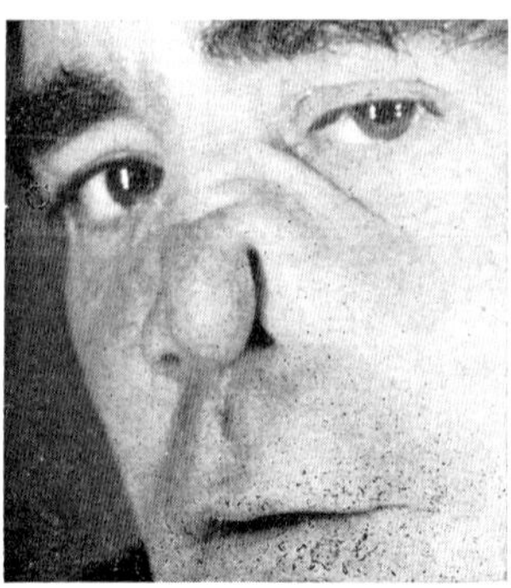

FIG. 68.

Gummatous destruction of ala nasi.

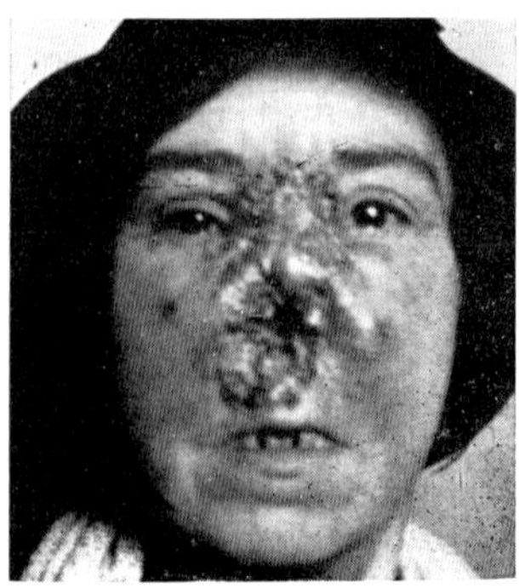

FIG. 69.

Widespread facial gummous destruction.

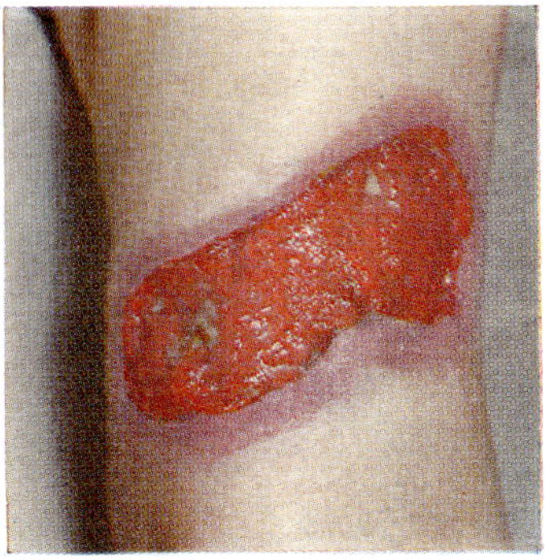

FIG. 70.

Gummatous ulcer of thigh involving deeper tissues.

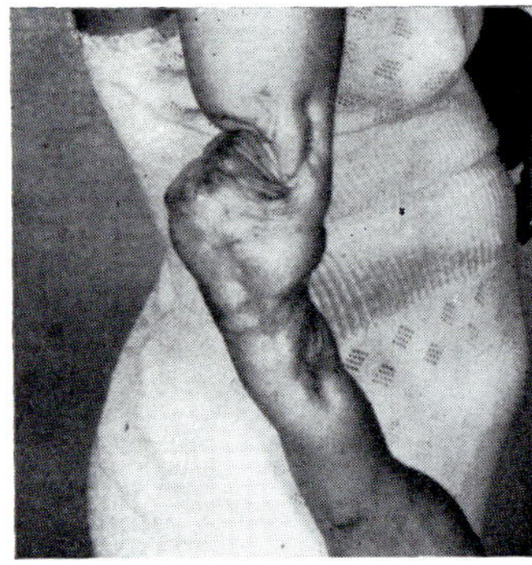

FIG. 71.

Results of extensive gummatous ulceration and destruction of the right arm.

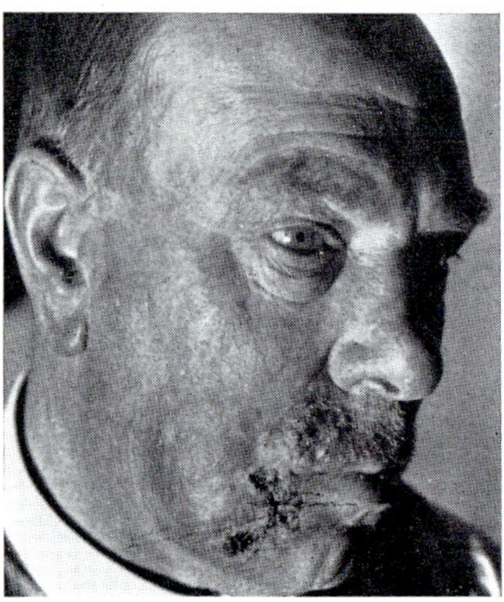

FIG. 72.

Subcutaneous gumma of the right cheek.

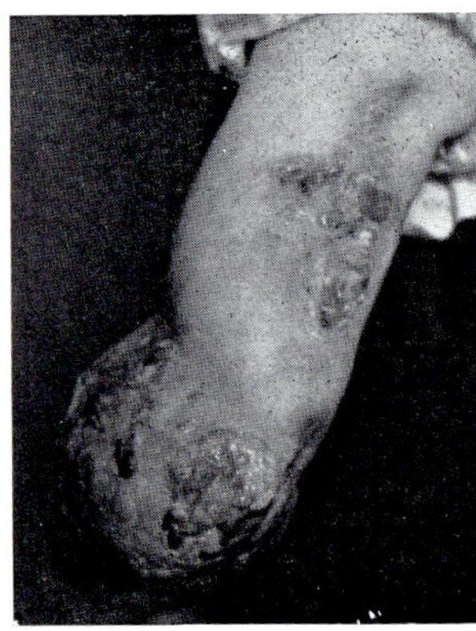

FIG. 73.

Gummous ulceration of triceps and at region of elbow.

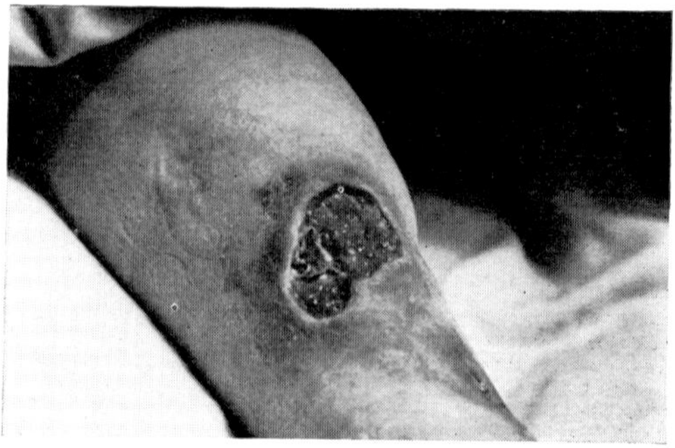

FIG. 74.
Typical punched-out gummous ulceration of leg.

for example the periosteum of the long bones. Central softening occurs, the gumma becomes adherent to the skin and breaks down, forming an ulcer with vertical 'punched-out' edges, sharply defined circular or kidney-shaped border and a base covered with exudate, a 'wash-leather' slough. The skin surrounding the ulcer may be normal in appearance, or may show a reddish or purplish discoloration. The gumma is usually solitary, but clusters of gummata can occur in the same areas, leading to polycyclic skin ulcerations. The destruction of deep tissue is often considerable following gummatous ulceration. Gummatous syphilides may occur anywhere in the body, the commonest sites being the upper part of the lower leg, the face, trunk, arms and scalp.

DIAGNOSIS

Gummata before ulceration must be differentiated from the various conditions which give rise to subcutaneous nodules: sebaceous cysts, lipomata fibromata, and, infrequently, from sarcomata, and erythema induratum (Bazin's disease); after ulceration, from tuberculous ulcers, malignant disease, varicose ulcers, actinomycosis, etc.

Mucous Membrane Lesions (localised or diffuse)

Infiltrations, corresponding to the nodular cutaneous syphilides, involve the mucous membranes, especially those of the tongue, the hard and soft palate, the lips, the tonsils and the pharynx. These infiltrations may not ulcerate, but give rise to sclerotic patches. Should they break down, they cause superficial ulcerations followed by flat reticulated irregular cicatrices. *Gummata* occur in the sub-mucous tissues, on the underlying periosteum or bone. The hard palate is especially liable to involvement. The gumma gives rise to the typical symptomless swelling, followed by central softening and ulceration leading to bone necrosis and perforation of the palate. *Interstitial sclerotic* lesions commonly affect the tongue, less frequently the lips, or other areas of the buccal mucosa, and may be either superficial or deep. In the early stages the tongue is red, swollen and glazed. As a result of cicatricial contracture, superficial furrowing or deep fissuring of the tongue becomes more pronounced, leading to distortion and fibrous contracture. Lymphatic obstruction may result in macroglossia.

The common sequel to interstitial glossitis is *leucoplakia*, which occurs characteristically on the dorsum or lateral surfaces of the tongue, and on the buccal mucosa at the tooth line. Leucoplakia is not necessarily a manifestation of syphilis but rather a protective tissue reaction to chronic irritation. Apart from syphilis, important causal factors are alcohol, tobacco, spices and dental irritation. The prominent symptom is local sensitiveness. The early appearance of leucoplakia is slight 'pearling' of the epithelium; when well-developed, white, thickened plaques are found.

DIAGNOSIS AND PROGNOSIS

Leucoplakia has to be differentiated from the mucous patches or moist papules of *early* syphilis, from the oral lesions of lichen planus and from thrush. In the treatment of leucoplakia, control of all sources of local irritation is essential. Slow symptomatic improvement follows antisyphilitic therapy, but the local condition

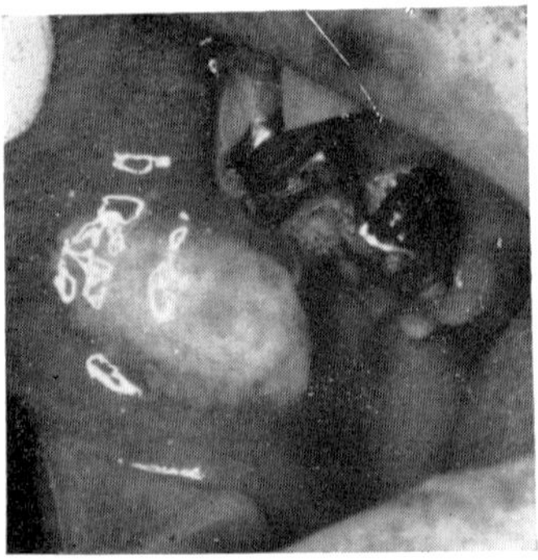

FIG. 75.

Gummatous late syphilide of buccal epithelium with ulceration.

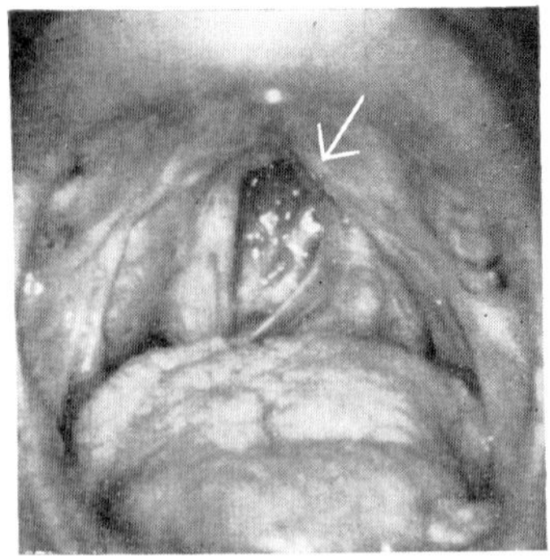

FIG. 76.

Results of gumma of the hard palate; large hole leading into the naso-pharynx.

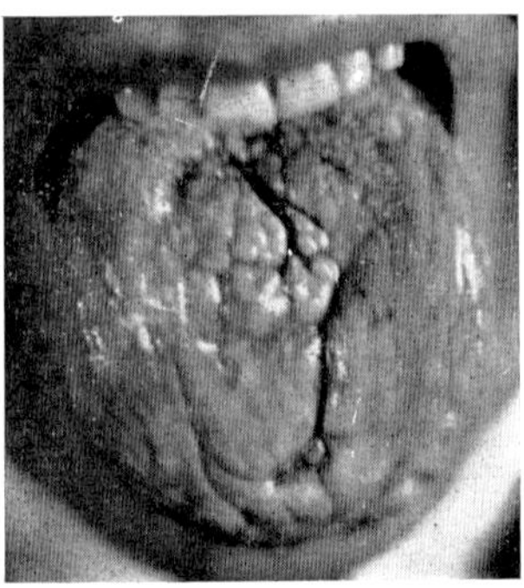

FIG. 77.

Chronic interstitial glossitis, showing marked fissuring and lobulation of the tongue.

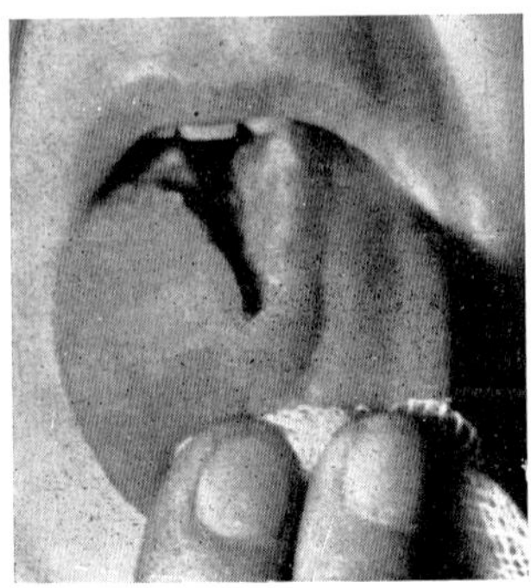

FIG. 78.

Gummous ulcer of the dorsum of the tongue.

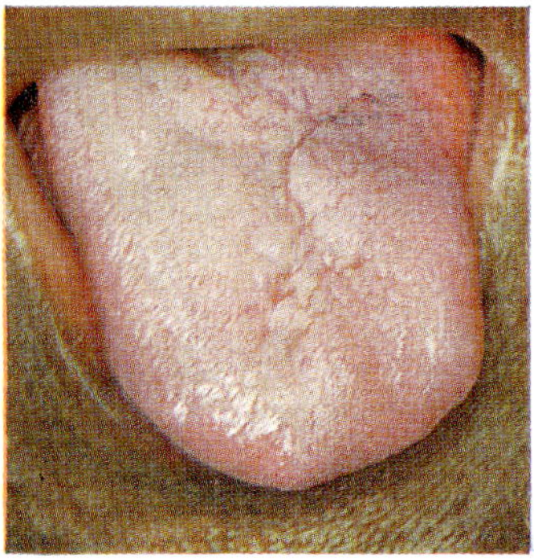

FIG. 79.
Syphilitic superficial glossitis and leukoplakia.

often remains apparently unaltered. Leucoplakia must be regarded as a pre-cancerous condition.

Lesions of Bones and Joints

In late syphilis bone and joint lesions run a slow course, and are associated with permanent changes in the bones affected. They are uncommon today. There is no basic difference between the pathological changes underlying syphilis of the bone and syphilis of other structures. The same changes occur, leading to localised or diffuse granulomatous tissue or gummatous infiltration, with new bone formation or, less frequently, rarefaction. The bones most commonly affected are, in order of frequency, the tibia, the nasal and palatal bones, the cranial bones, the femur, the humerus and the patella.

BONES

Classification according to the structures involved:—

1. Ostealgia (osteocopic pains)
2. Periostitis
3. Osteitis (panosteitis or osteomyelitis)
4. Gumma of bone

(2–4: Localised or diffuse)

1. *Ostealgia* varies in degree from a slight dull ache up to the most excruciating lancinating pains, usually intermittent, not infrequently migratory, and presenting periodic nocturnal exacerbations which interfere with rest. No local abnormalities are detected on clinical or X-ray examination. Salicylates fail to afford relief, but specific treatment is rapidly effective.

2. *Periostitis* causes pain of a similar nature where the changes consist at first of periosteal thickening, causing tender areas.

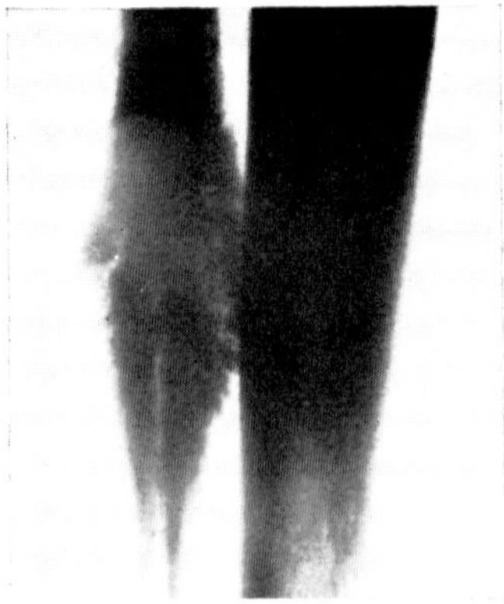

FIG. 80.

Syphilitic osteo-periostitis of fibula, the changes suggesting osteogenic sarcoma.

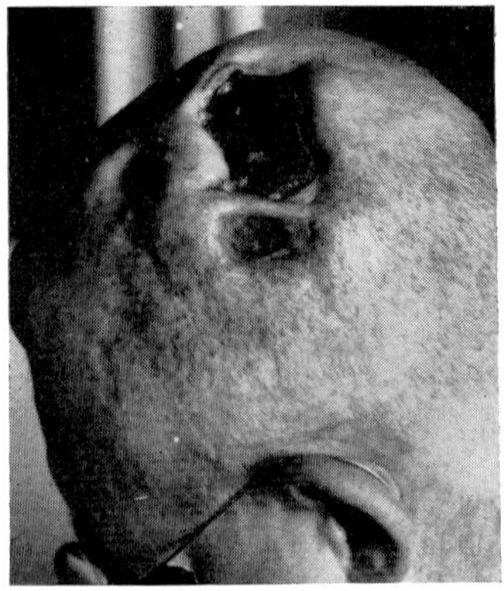

FIG. 81.

Syphilitic osteitis of skull, showing sequestrum formation of outer table. Healed nodular cutaneous lesions are present on the cheek.

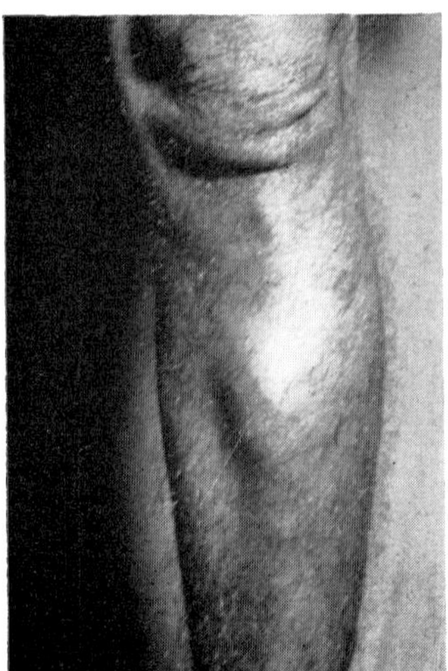

FIG. 82.

Gumma of tibia.

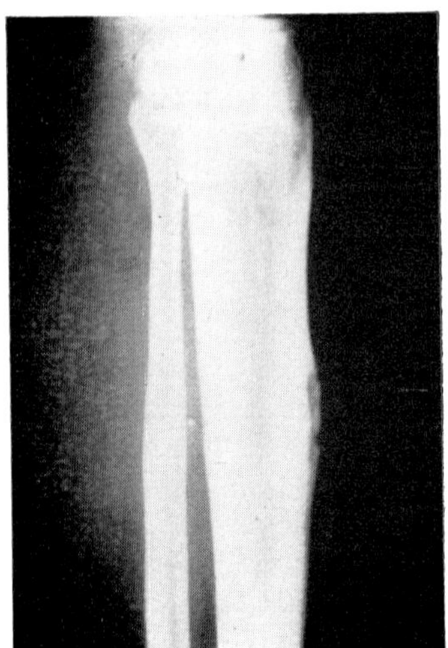

FIG. 83.

X-ray of (Fig. 80) showing periosteal thickening together with boney destruction.

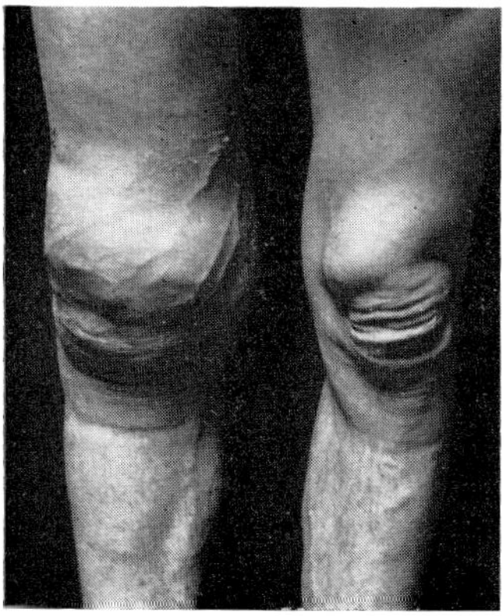

FIG. 84.

Charcot's disease of the knee joint, showing marked swelling and dilatation of the superficial veins.

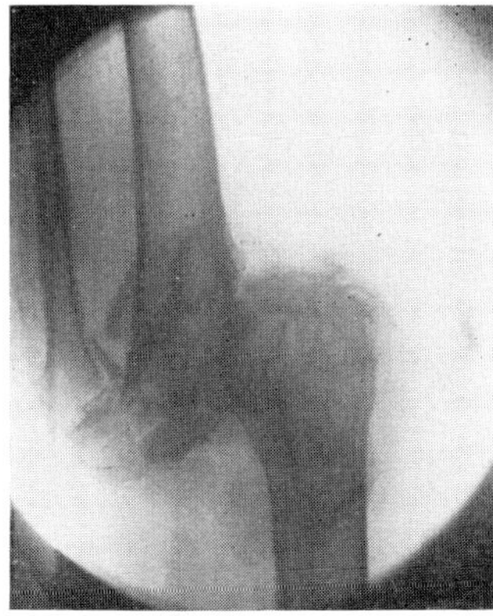

FIG. 85.

Destruction of knee joint due to Charcot's arthropathy.

Later sub-periosteal deposition of new bone gives rise to localised or diffuse bony thickening, which should be differentiated from osteogenic sarcoma.

3. *Osteitis* is localised or diffuse. In localised osteitis initial osteosclerosis is followed by osteoporosis which may result in pathological fracture. Diffuse osteitis invariably causes sclerotic changes, leading to increased circumference, size and density of the bone. The tibia and femur are most commonly affected, giving rise in the former to the 'sabre blade' deformity. This is more frequently met with in congenital syphilis. Sequestrum and sinus formation are rare. It has to be distinguished from osteitis deformans and tuberculous osteitis.

Syphilitic *dactylitis* occurs both in congenital and acquired syphilis. It is a pan-osteitis and begins as a firm, painless, flask-shaped bony swelling covered by normal or slightly reddened skin. It affects the phalanges, less frequently the metacarpals and metatarsals. Pain is absent. Syphilitic dactylitis may remain apparently stationary for several months, tending ultimately to spontaneous resolution, leaving a shortened phalanx. Sequestrum or sinus formation is not infrequent.

4. *Gummatous* osteitis and osteomyelitis are very rare, appearing as a combination of proliferative and destructive changes. Surrounding tissues are usually involved.

Joints

Disorders can be classified as:—

1. Arthralgia 2. Synovitis 3. Hydrarthrosis	in early and late syphilis
4. Osteochondroarthropathy 5. Gummatous perisynovitis 6. Tabetic arthropathy (Charcot's joints)	in late syphilis.

1. *Arthralgia*, corresponding to ostealgia, especially in the large joints, is not accompanied by clinical or X-ray changes. Arthralgia may continue for long periods; specific treatment, however, rapidly brings an end to the symptoms.

2. *Synovitis* in its acute form is more commonly met with in early generalised syphilis and may be accompanied by pyrexia. In acute or chronic synovitis one or more of the large joints can be affected; infrequently the smaller joints. X-ray changes are absent. Specific treatment is followed by marked improvement.

3. *Hydrarthrosis* occurs in association with acute and subacute synovitis or may arise insiduously. In the latter type the larger joints are more commonly affected; frequently the condition is polyarticular. No changes, apart from swelling due to the accumulation of fluid, can be detected in the articular or periarticular structures on clinical or X-ray examination. Movement is limited by the effusion. The condition tends towards spontaneous remission and recurrence.

4. *Osteochondroarthropathy* generally involves one of the larger joints, commonly the knee or the elbow, and is frequently associated with gummatous osteomyelitis of the adjacent areas of long bone. The process is a combination of destructive and

proliferative changes affecting the articular cartilage and the underlying bone and the synovial structures, giving rise to a globular, distended, doughy joint (white swelling). Pain may be absent in the early stages, but becomes more prominent later. The skin over the joint is pale. The movements of the joint are less limited than expected. Specific treatment is followed by rapid movement.

5. *Gummatous perisynovitis* affects a large joint, there being synovial thickening accompanied by effusion. The condition is asymptomatic.

6. *Tabetic arthropathy* (*Charcot's joints*). Neurotrophic changes may affect the joints in tabes dorsalis. Usually one of the large joints, the knee, hip, shoulder or ankle, is affected; occasionally, however, multiple large or smaller joints may be involved. In the early stages exudation occurs into the joint cavity and peri-articular structures. This is followed by rapid, painless articular disorganisation, synovial thickening and villous formation, erosion of articular cartilage with eburnation or destruction of the underlying bone. Destruction of the ligaments gives rise to a painless flail joint. The X-ray appearances show gross disorganisation, disappearance of cartilage and articular margins of bone, and bony rarefaction. Frequently, in the final stages, portions of osseous tissue (sequestra) are lying free in and about the joint. After a few years a gradual improvement takes place with an increase in bone density. Deformity, however, remains permanent.

DIAGNOSIS

This is usually obvious. Syringomyelia or severe subacute combined degeneration, amongst other rarer disorders, can give rise to similar joint lesions.

Pathological fracture and perforating ulcer (trophic ulceration) not infrequently occur in tabes; the usual situation is the sole of the foot or one of the toes. The slow painless ulceration gradually extends down to the bone which may sequestrate or becomes carious. These ulcers are refractory to treatment. Similar conditions are occasionally found in diabetic peripheral neuritis.

Juxta-articular nodes are localised gummata, involving the joint capsule, bursae or tendon sheaths, which undergo fibrotic degeneration. They may give rise to a hard nodule attached for example to the extensor aspects of the joint capsule. Specific treatment may cause the nodes to resolve, or they can prove completely refractory.

Lesions of Muscle, Tendon and Bursa

In early generalised syphilis, *myalgia*, corresponding to arthralgia and ostealgia, may be noted. In late syphilis localised or diffuse *myositis* is also found. The onset is usually insidious, the patient experiencing infrequent cramps. There is limitation of extension of the affected muscle. Pain is marked and the muscle becomes progressively more hard. Considerable deformity can result, but the prognosis is good. Multiple *gummata* may arise in muscle. Tenosynovitis: as in secondary syphilis, serous tenosynovitis may occur later in the disease, commonly affecting the tendons on the dorsum of the wrist or on the anterior aspect of the ankle joint. Swelling is rapid and painless, and there is a creaking on movement, but movement itself is not interfered with. The skin is generally unaltered. Gummatous *tenosynovitis* commences as a localised or diffuse infiltration of the tendon sheath, forming an irregular lumpy swelling which becomes adherent to the skin, softens and ulcerates, leaving a chronic, often serpiginous, ulcer. Sloughing of the tendon may occur. Gummata also sometimes arise in the tendons. An indolent serous *bursitis* may occur at any time during the course of generalised syphilis. In late syphilis gummatous bursitis gradually leads to the formation of a solid tumour which later may ulcerate.

TREATMENT OF LATE SYPHILIS

See Treatment of Cardiovascular Syphilis (p. 70) etc.

Cardiovascular Syphilis

Syphilis is fundamentally a disease of blood vessels (p. 25). It is not surprising therefore to find important manifestations

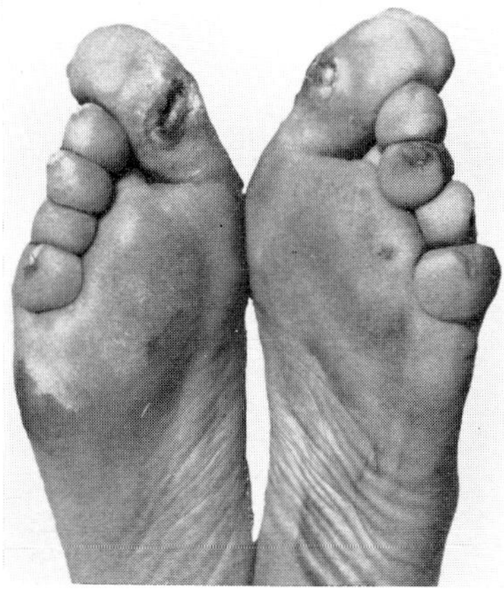

FIG. 86.
Perforating ulcers in tabes dorsalis.

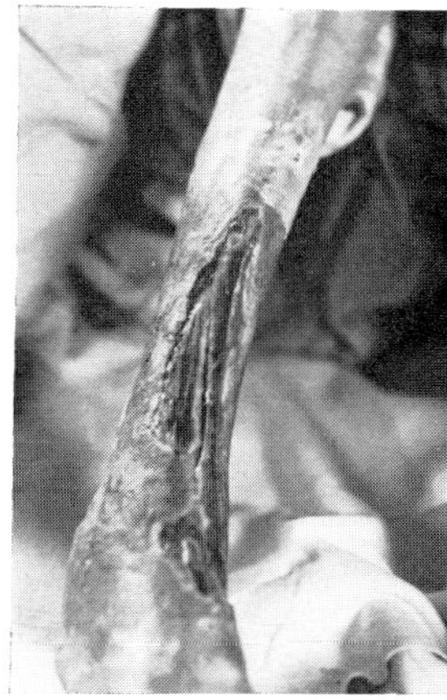

FIG. 87.
Gummatous tenosynovitis in the ulcerative stage.

related to the cardiovascular system, all the elements of which are affected during the generalised stage of the disease. Symptoms or signs develop infrequently during the secondary stage. It is usual, however, to find that localising cardiovascular symptoms appear after an insiduous onset varying in length from 10 to 30 years after infection. Rarely, this can occur after only a few years.

Syphilitic involvement of the heart and blood vessels may be classified as:—

1. Syphilis of the small and medium sized vessels.
2. Syphilis of the aorta and heart.

Syphilis of the Small and Medium-Sized Vessels

Although specific lesions in late syphilis are related to the small blood vessels, localised manifestations of syphilitic affection of small arteries or veins are rarely met with today. They may occur as nodular thickenings along a vein, with evidence of periphlebitis or an erythema nodosum-like eruption. Occasionally symptoms of vascular disturbance occur simulating Raynaud's or Buerger's disease. Aneurisms of the smaller and medium sized arteries occasionally arise in such positions as the popliteal artery, where traumatic factors may play a part.

Syphilis of the Aorta and Heart

Aortitis is more common in men than in women, 80 per cent of cases being recognised in the former sex. Heavy exertion may be one determining factor. The granulomatous syphilitic changes begin in the vasa vasorum of the tunica media of the first part of the aorta, and result in fragmentation or complete loss of elastic and muscular coats and their replacement by fibrous tissue. The incomplete contraction of this tissue leads to depressed linear or stellate scars. The intima shows compensatory thickening, but can appear unaltered. The fibrous tissue in syphilis is thin and gradually stretches, leading progressively to aortic dilatation and aneurysm, and dilatation of the aortic ring. Incompetence of the aortic valve results from a weak, dilated aortic ring and possibly from adhesions along the valve cusps. Clinically we are able to recognise: (1) aortitis; (2) aortitis with aortic incompetence; (3) aortitis with aneurysm formation; (4) aortitis with myocardial ischaemia; or combinations of these groups. Aortic stenosis, in the opinion of most authorities, is said not to occur in syphilis.

SYMPTOMS

In the early stages the symptoms may be vague and not directly indicative of the cardiovascular lesion. Headache, often of a throbbing character, attacks of giddiness, faintness on rising or stooping, irritability or defects of memory may be complained of. Palpitation and vague anginal pains occur on exertion or at rest. As the underlying aortic changes become more marked, the symptoms become more severe and localising. Precordial or substernal pain of either constant dull or sharp severe character occurs and may radiate to the scapula or down the arm. Characteristically such substernal pain is usually not closely related to exertion, and is present also at night. Nocturnal dyspnoea and orthopnoea, and oedema of the feet, progressively appear as left ventricular failure is followed by right ventricular failure.

The earliest physical sign of aortitis is an accentuation of the aortic second sound, with or without an aortic systolic murmur. When aortic incompetence occurs, more definite clinical signs appear: cardiac murmurs, in particular a soft blowing diastolic murmur over the aortic area, and conducted down the left side of the sternum, appearing also in the mitral area (Austin Flint), marked cardiac enlargement, collapsing pulse, capillary pulsation and increased pulse pressure as noted by the raised systolic and depressed diastolic blood pressure. X-ray examination shows characteristic broadening of the ascending aorta and arch.

Aortic Aneurysm.

The signs and symptoms vary according to whether the sinuses of Valsalva, the ascending, transverse or descending portion of the aortic arch are involved. Aneurysmal dilatation of the *sinuses of Valsalva* at first may be asymptomatic, then give rise to symptoms and signs of myocardial ischaemia with or without those of a co-existing aortic incompetence.

Aneurysm of the *ascending aortic arch* gives rise to anginal pain, and, if the aneurysm be saccular, to a brassy paroxysmal cough. The physical signs are those of an expansile pulsating tumour to the right of the sternum. A systolic thrill and murmur occur over the sac, the aortic second sound is accentuated, or if there is incompetence it is replaced by a murmur. The heart is frequently displaced to the left. The pupils are often unequal, due to sympathetic nerve involvement. Pressure on the recurrent laryngeal nerve leads to paralysis of the right vocal cord with alteration of the voice (Horner's syndrome).

Aneurysm of the *transverse aortic arch* more commonly gives rise to alterations of voice, and frequently to paroxysmal brassy cough, inequality of the pupils, laryngeal paralysis, tracheal tug and suprasternal pulsation. If the aneurysmal sac is directed downwards compression of the left bronchus results in signs of bronchiectasis, bronchopneumonia or collapse of the lung.

Aneurysm of the *descending arch* may give rise to few symptoms other than those of pressure on the lung structures, vertebrae or ribs. A pulsating tumour may be present in the left interscapular space.

Coronary Ostial Stenosis

Sclerosis or partial occlusion of the mouths of the coronary arteries is not uncommonly associated with aortic valve disease or aneurysm. Anginal attacks become frequent.

Syphilis of the Myocardium

Myocardial disturbances may occur in *early* syphilis, the diagnosis depending on the rapid onset of the cardiac symptoms in the course of early generalised infection. It is confirmed by the prompt symptomatic relief following specific therapy. In the *late* stages of syphilis, myocardial changes follow ostial stenosis, coronary arteritis or, occasionally, gummatous myocarditis. These changes are: interstitial fibrosis and degeneration of the heart muscle or, rarely, gumma. The symptoms are those of a slowly progressive myocardial insufficiency. The electrocardiogram sometimes demonstrates such features as a bundle branch block.

DIAGNOSIS AND PROGNOSIS

Routine X-ray examination in late syphilis may demonstrate early aortic widening before clinical signs can be detected. The specific serum tests are invariably positive in active disease, when the E.S.R. also is frequently raised.

The early detection of syphilitic aortitis improves the prospect of arrest of the disease. The more advanced the physical changes the less favourable is the outlook, the expectation of life varying from six months to several years, on average five years in a moderately severe case.

TREATMENT

The treatment varies according to the stage of the syphilis when cardiovascular symptoms occur, its activity and its extent. In the

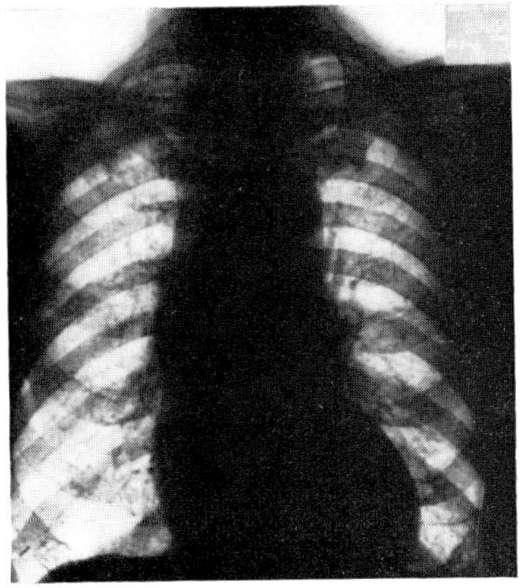

FIG. 88.

Early stages of aortitis, showing widening of the ascending aorta.

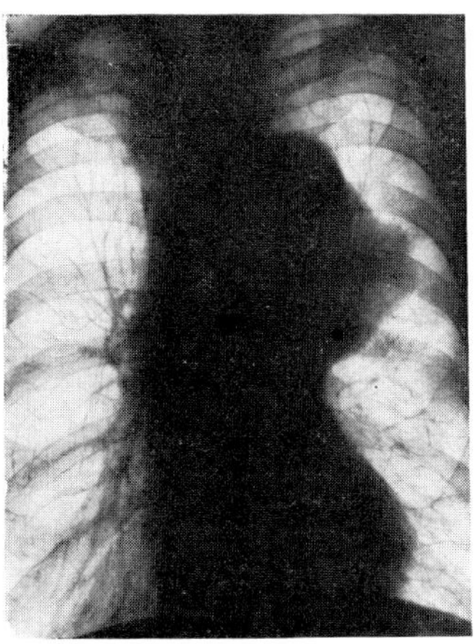

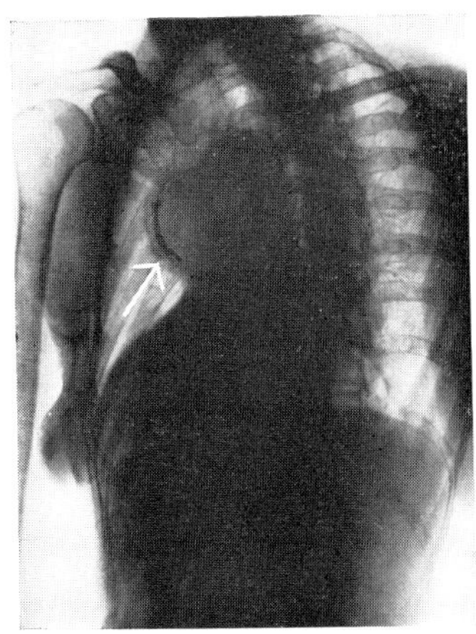

FIG. 89*a*. FIG. 89*b*.

Aortic aneurysm, demonstrating diagnostic linear calcification in the aortic well.

late stages it must be remembered that a varying degree of fibrous replacement of the muscular and elastic structures has already occurred, and, while it is possible to obtain symptomatic relief, it is impossible to reconstitute the normal anatomical structure of the parts. Every effort must, however, be made to arrest the inflammatory and degenerative processes and to secure for the individual the maximal clinical improvement. The general principles are: (1) rest in bed, the administration of digitalis or other cardiac drugs according to standard medical practice; (2) the administration of potassium iodide in dosage of 2·0–2·6 g. t.d.s. for a period of two weeks; (3) the use of steroid therapy for two to three days to protect the patient from a hyper-sensitivity reaction (Jarisch-Herxheimer): for example prednisolone 20 mg. daily by mouth in divided dosage for three days, unless there are contraindications, first reducing then tailing off the drug after antibiotic therapy has been started; and (4) administration of *penicillin* or other antibiotic.

The aim of antibiotic treatment is to eradicate the treponeme and obtain the greatest possible restoration to normal of the affected tissues, with the minimal formation of scar tissue. In late syphilis, therapy may on rare occasions result in a paradox: a rapid healing, by conversion of the syphilitic infiltration into contractile scar tissue, may lead in certain situations to destruction of the parenchyma of an organ (*e.g.* the liver by cirrhotic changes, or in the case of an artery, for example the coronary, by complete occlusion). Thus, after a brief period of symptomatic improvement, there is an irreversible deterioration in the condition of the patient. In late syphilis, this reaction may be exacerbated by tissue destruction following a Herxheimer reaction, and can be largely avoided by the use of corticosteroids before starting antibiotic therapy.

Penicillin should be administered in high doses in cardiovascular syphilis. It is recommended that 1·0 mega-unit of procaine penicillin G, or benzathine penicillin, fortified by 1·0 mega-unit of benzyl penicillin should be injected daily, for three weeks. Retreatment courses of two to three weeks' duration using larger doses should be given to the patient at an interval of six months to a year or two, depending upon the clinical condition and the serological titres.

In late syphilis of other varieties, excepting neurosyphilis, it is not necessary to resort to such large amounts of antibiotic therapy. A two-week course of 1·0 mega-unit of procaine penicillin injected daily, followed by observation of the patient and of the serological titres, is often sufficient.

Tetracycline may be administered to the patient who is sensitive to penicillin. This drug must be used in relatively large doses, that is, 2 to 3 g. a day (given six-hourly in divided dosage) for two or three weeks at a time. Nystatin, 0·5 mega-unit t.d.s., has to be taken by mouth when alimentary candidasis becomes troublesome in those taking tetracycline. Erythromycin may not be entirely satisfactory. *Cephaloridine* can be given intramuscularly 2·0 g. daily.

Assessment of clinical progress is made after a course of treatment is completed, and management maintained to secure the maximum of improvement, always bearing in mind that in cardiovascular syphilis comparatively large courses of specific treatment are advisable.*

Other lesions of Viscera

LIVER

Single or multiple gumma occasionally arise, or a diffuse gummatous infiltration, leading to cirrhotic changes. Fibrosis with great distortion of the shape of the organ can occur. Portal cirrhosis, tumours, parasitic disease or cholelithiasis are suggested. Amyloid changes can follow.

Gummata are rarely to be found in the stomach, pancreas or intestines. There may be marked fibrous thickening known as a syphiloma, especially in the rectum; it is to be distinguished from lymphogranuloma, regional ileitis and malignant disease. Gummata or perisplenitis may occur in the spleen.

A slight degree of microcytic anaemia is common in late syphilis. Paroxysmal haemoglobinuria is rarely seen and is less

* Note under Serology and Treatment of fixed high titres.

common in late acquired than in congenital syphilis. There occurs fever and prostration, with haemoglobinuria on warming after a slight chill, due to the presence of 'cold' haemolysin.

The enlargement of the lymph nodes, due to gummatous changes in late syphilis, may affect a solitary gland or a group of glands.

Renal gumma is rare.

Endocrine Glands

Involvement of thyroid, thymus, supra-renals or pituitary is very rare, and proof that syphilis is responsible is difficult to find. The therapeutic test—that is, a favourable response to specific treatment—is the only available clinical evidence for it. Damage occurs either through diffuse gummatous infiltration or gummata.

RESPIRATORY TRACT

Late syphilis of the larynx can present as a diffuse gummatous infiltration; a solitary gumma leads to ulceration, or to a perichondritis of the arytenoid cartilage. Contracture and stenosis may result from the first. Syphilis, in contrast to tuberculosis, is painless: a response to specific treatment will distinguish between syphilis and malignant disease.

Syphilis of the lungs and bronchi is extremely rare. Gummata have been described in the hilar regions with appearance on X-ray, and should be diagnosed only after careful consideration of all other possible causes, and a favourable response to specific treatment.

Genito-Urinary Organs

In late syphilis both gummatous infiltrations and isolated gummata are rarely to be seen in the kidney, bladder and prostate. Gumma of testis is less rare. The testicular sensation is lost; there is often a small hydrocoele, and the organ feels heavy. The lesion may break down and ulceration occur. Although the epididymis may be involved in this spread, it is primarily affected by such infections as tuberculosis and gonorrhoea, whereas the testis is affected by mumps (which is often bilateral) and in malignant disease. Uterus, salpinges and ovaries are also rarely involved, in the same manner as the male generative organs.

The Eye

Affections in late syphilis are most commonly due to choroiditis, which presents as yellow-greyish foci of inflammation in the fundus, deep to the retinal vessels. Choroiditis of the 'spidery' type can also occur. Small diffuse opacities may be present in the posterior portion of the vitreous. Such lesions in the choroid must be distinguished from those of toxoplasmosis, retinitis pigmentosa and other causes of choroido-retinitis. Optic neuritis is not infrequent in neurosyphilis. When this occurs posteriorly, leading to early atrophy, the condition is known as *primary optic atrophy*. Interstitial keratitis, an inflammation of the deep layer of the cornea, is relatively common in congenital syphilis (p. 90).

The Ear

Acquired syphilis rarely affects the *internal ear*. Occasional temporary loss of hearing due to hyperaemia in the *early* infectious stage soon passes off. In late syphilis otosclerosis and labyrinthitis may result in deafness and Ménière's syndrome. If gummatous meningitis involves the eighth cranial nerve, deafness ensues. The prognosis is good only if the conditions are treated early.

Neurosyphilis

Syphilis was at one time one of the most important causes of organic disease of the central nervous system. After early generalisation of the infection there is a likelihood of involvement of the meninges, blood vessels or parenchyma of the brain or spinal cord. Symptoms and signs of neurosyphilis may appear before, or concurrently with, the appearance of the general skin eruption; more commonly, however, their onset occurs after an interval varying from one to fifteen years, or even more. During the latent period vague symptoms arise: neurasthenia with headache, dizziness, anorexia, etc., not directly suggestive of neurosyphilis. Failure to consider this possibility, and to examine the CSF at this stage, may result in irreparable tissue destruction before the true diagnosis is arrived at.

Neurosyphilis may be classified as:—

1. Meningovascular—
   (*a*) Mainly meningeal:—cerebral; meningitis (basal or of the convexity): spinal; hypertrophic pachymeningitis, and meningomyelitis.
   (*b*) Mainly vascular:—cerebral: spinal; 'myelitis'; and that caused by thrombotic lesions.
2. Parenchymatous—
   Syphilitic paresis (G.P.I.); tabes dorsalis; tabo-paresis; midbrain involvement; cord syndromes.
3. Gumma formation.
4. Peripheral nerve involvement.
5. Asymptomatic neurosyphilis.

PATHOLOGY

The underlying pathological changes are invariably more diffuse than is suggested by the signs and symptoms, and in many cases more than one group of structures is involved. The pathological basis of neurosyphilis is similar to that in other tissues. Obliterative endarteritis takes place with perivascular small, round cell and plasma cell infiltration leading to meningeal thickening, and progressively to impaired nutrition, chromatolysis, vacuolation and ultimately complete destruction of the parenchymal cells with increase of interstitial tissue.

Meningovascular Syphilis

Meningeal

In the majority of cases the basal meninges are affected. Early or late syphilitic meningeal involvement may be asymptomatic: more commonly, however, headache of varying severity, insomnia, slight dizziness, general lassitude, inability to concentrate or perform routine tasks or nervous irritability are complained of. Paralyses are common; the third, fourth, sixth, and occasionally the seventh cranial nerves may be involved. Monoplegias, paraplegias or epileptiform seizures occur. Syphilis of the spinal meninges gives rise to both localised and diffuse motor symptoms and sensory symptoms.

DIAGNOSIS AND PROGNOSIS

Meningeal syphilis has to be distinguished from functional nervous disorders, such as neurasthenia or neurosis, and from the early stages of organic disease, for example disseminated sclerosis, chronic meningitis or tumours. The examination of the spinal fluid is conclusive (p. 193). The response to treatment is usually good; symptoms are relieved and the cerebro-spinal fluid rapidly becomes normal.

Vascular

Involvement of the cerebrospinal blood vessels may occur at any stage in the course of generalised syphilis. The clinical picture depends upon the degree of vascular occlusion, from thrombosis or from haemorrhage into the brain or cord substance. The symptoms are at first mild and transitory, becoming increasingly more severe: headache, vertigo, progressive loss of mental powers and transient paralyses. Later a definite clinical picture (monoplegia, paraplegia or hemiplegia) develops, often without loss of consciousness or loss of control of the sphincters. Rupture of a vessel may cause sudden death. Aneurysm formation may affect the circle of Willis.

DIAGNOSIS AND PROGNOSIS

The occurrence of cerebrovascular phenomena in an adult, often under the age of forty years, and the absence of evidence of peripheral vascular disease should suggest the possibility of a syphilitic cause. Generalised cerebral arterio-sclerosis rarely occurs at this age. The cerebrospinal fluid may show few abnormalities. Usually, however, the cell count is raised, the globulin content is increased, the Wassermann reaction is positive and the gold-sol reaction shows a luetic curve (p. 80).

In partial paralysis due to incomplete vascular occlusion spontaneous recovery may ensue. The condition clears up rapidly under treatment. When haemorrhage or thrombosis has occurred, recovery is more complete than in cases due to a *non*-syphilitic cause.

Myelitis

Syphilitic myelitis is rare and due to a combination of meningomyelitis and thrombosis. Two types occur: an *acute transverse myelitis* of rapid onset, frequently without preceding motor or sensory irritation. The symptoms depend upon the level of the cord at which the lesion occurs. Generally there is complete paralysis from the pelvis downwards with alteration or complete loss of sensation. The temperature sense may remain unimpaired. A chronic meningomyelitis is more common and results in an incomplete transverse lesion. The dorsal area is most commonly affected, giving rise to vague pains in the back and limbs, paraesthesia and motor weakness. Spastic paraplegia may result. Sensory changes are similar to those found in acute myelitis. The tendon reflexes are usually exaggerated and bladder disturbances are common. *Erb's* syphilitic spinal paralysis and syphilitic *amyotrophy* is only one stage in a slow progressive syphilitic meningomyelitis (p. 79).

Parenchymatous Neurosyphilis

Syphilitic Paresis (General Paralysis of the Insane; Dementia Paralytica)

The onset of paresis occurs at any time after infection, the usual interval being 10 to 15 years. Men are more commonly affected than women. The initial symptoms are frequently vague and indefinite, the individual being apparently neurasthenic, or complaining of headaches, insomnia, inability to concentrate, absent-mindedness or depression. Irritability, intemperance, extravagance and deterioration of personal habits may cause the patient's relatives to seek advice. There is difficulty in association of ideas, and a loss of memory for recent events; the features of an organic dementia.

CLINICAL FEATURES

These are: (1) progressive *mental impairment*, delusions and depression. (2) *Convulsive seizures*: the patient has a fit and becomes unconscious, remaining so for periods varying from a few hours to a day or two: these attacks may suggest uraemia, diabetic coma or cerebrovascular accident. (3) *Speech* is thick and slurred, syllables being missed out and the consonants running together: *tremors* of the lips and tongue are observed during articulation: the handwriting may show characteristic changes due to muscular tremor: familiar words are mis-spelt or omitted. (4) Physical signs are few and in the early stages may be absent: irregularity of the pupils and a sluggish reaction to light, fine tremor of the muscles of the face, tongue or hands or a 'trombone tremor' of the tongue may be present. The tendon reflexes can be normal but usually are exaggerated. Later, inequality in size of the pupils, loss of pupillary light reaction with retention of accommodation (Argyll Robertson), marked exaggeration of the tendon reflexes and an *extensor plantar* reflex may be found.

DIAGNOSIS AND PROGNOSIS

Syphilitic paresis has to be distinguished from neurosis, chronic alcoholism, psychotic depression, neurasthenia, intracranial tumours, from generalised arterio-sclerosis and presenile dementia. These conditions may be excluded on clinical grounds, by the absence of the serological reactions associated with syphilis and by the changes in the cerebrospinal fluid (p. 80). Confirmation of the diagnosis of syphilitic paresis indicates a serious prognosis. If the patient is left untreated there is rapidly progressive mental and physical deterioration leading to death within a few years. Spontaneous remissions, which may last for periods varying from a few weeks to several months, are not uncommon, the patient appearing 'normal'. But the symptoms eventually recur. In general, the earlier the condition is detected and the less marked the mental and physical changes, the better is the outlook. Alterations in speech or advanced mental changes are of grave import. Thorough treatment in early stages promises a relatively good prognosis. Patients with a permanent mental deficit are better able to adjust to life after treatment, if they can retain a close relationship with their previous social environment and occupation.

TABES DORSALIS (Locomotor Ataxia)

The pathology of tabes dorsalis is essentially a posterior root ganglionitis due to a pia-arachnoiditis, with degeneration of the sensory columns of the lower levels of the spinal cord. There are also pathological changes in the brain as shown by the frequency of optic atrophy, pupillary changes and cranial nerve pareses. It is unusual for the condition to be diagnosed at a very early stage; more often the disease has been present a number of years before symptoms bring the patient to a doctor. The early features of tabes show considerable variation. In some cases failing vision, in others inability to walk or lightening pains may first call attention to the underlying condition.

The cardinal symptoms and signs suggesting the diagnosis are:—

1. *Loss of tendon reflexes.* Knee and ankle jerks are lost early in the course of tabes. The superficial reflexes may be lost later.

2. *Ocular changes.* In the early stages the pupils react sluggishly to light; later Argyll-Robertson pupils develop: complete loss of reaction to light, with retention of that to accommodation; the pupils are frequently small (myosis), unequal in size and show irregularity in outline, with incomplete reaction to mydriatics. *Optic atrophy*, progressing to complete loss of vision in three to five years, unilateral or bilateral *ptosis*, or *ocular pareses* may be the earliest sign.

3. *Sensory changes.* The patient first notices difficulty in walking in the dark or in balancing with the eyes shut (*e.g.* when washing the face). Later, difficulty is experienced in going up or down stairs or over uneven ground. The gait becomes characteristic: the feet wide apart, raised high, thrown forward, hyper-extending the knee, and brought down with a stamping motion (ataxia). *Romberg's sign* is positive which is a sign of posterior column ataxia with muscular hypotonia and incoordination: the

patient sways and shows a marked tendency to fall when asked to stand with the toes and heels together and the eyes closed. *Lightning pains* are sharp pains, frequently stabbing, of short duration, referred commonly to the sciatic distribution. Attacks occur at irregular intervals, varying from a few hours to several weeks, and become increasingly severe. Prolonged pains of 'rheumatic' character are not uncommon. *Girdle pains* produce a feeling of painful constriction of the chest or waist. *Visceral crises*: violent attacks of pain referred to the stomach, the larynx, the urinary bladder or pelvis of the kidney occur, and are associated with nausea and vomiting. The temperature is not raised. According to the level involved, appendicitis, biliary and renal colic, or gastric perforation may be suggested. Areas of anaesthesia to *light touch* occur bilaterally, especially on the face, chest and ankles. Diminution in superficial pain sense affects the legs or trunk. *Deep sensibility* in bones and tendons is impaired. *Visceral analgesia* may, rarely, occur through involvement of the spinal sympathetic afferent nerves, and mask an abdominal lesion.

4. *Sphincters.* Dysfunction of the bladder sphincter is common, leading first to delay and difficulty in micturition, 'stammering' micturition, and later retention with overflow incontinence. This is followed by cystitis and ascending urinary infection. Impotence is common. Sexual desire and response are lost.

5. *Trophic lesions.* Perforating ulcers, commonly affecting the ball of the great toe, arthropathies (Charcot's Joint), pathological fractures, and muscular wasting not infrequently occur.

6. *Mental powers* show no impairment in tabes.

DIAGNOSIS AND PROGNOSIS

Tabes must be differentiated from peripheral neuritis following poisoning (*e.g.* alcohol, arsenic), diphtheria, diabetes, etc.; from organic diseases the symptoms of which may be suggested by the pain of visceral crises; from causes of ataxia such as cerebellar lesions; and from diseases affecting the long tracts of the spinal cord, for example disseminated sclerosis, syringomyelia, and subacute combined degeneration. The history, pupillary signs, and other clinical findings should indicate the possibility of tabes. Confirmation of the diagnosis is made by serological examinations of the blood and cerebrospinal fluid. On the other hand, in a case of several years' duration the serological tests may be negative and the cerebrospinal fluid normal (p. 80). Syphilitic meningomyelitis may closely simulate tabes: but this condition occurs earlier, progress is more rapid, and recovery under treatment is speedier and complete. The course of untreated tabes is unpredictable: the condition may progress rapidly to complete paralysis and fatal issue from urinary or other intercurrent infection, or it may be arrested at any stage. Progression may occur after remissions lasting many years, and takes place despite treatment. The earlier the diagnosis of tabes dorsalis is made and treatment is instituted, the better is the outlook for arrest of the disease. Complete recovery never occurs, but stabilisation is possible often with considerable physical improvement.

Midbrain Syphilis, Amytrophy and Chronic Spinal Cord Syndromes

Muscular hypertonia and tremors of *Parkinsonian* type have been described in association with Tabes dorsalis. The prognosis is said to be better than in paralysis agitans.

Cerebrospinal syphilis as a chronic spinal malady may affect the anterior horn cells, either due to inflammation of the meningeal sheaths of the spinal nerve roots, or as a result of meningomyelitis. Occasionally it causes primary degeneration. A *progressive muscular atrophy* results.

Lateral sclerosis may occur alone (*Erb's*) or combined with signs of tabes. The signs are those of an upper motor neurone paraplegia; spastic gait, increased lower limb deep reflexes, absent abdominal, and extensor plantar responses.

Optic atrophy in syphilis is usually progressive if the condition has reached a point of low visual acuity prior to treatment. It is due to degeneration of the optic nerve, as featured by the pallor of the whole optic disc, in syphilis the colour being often greyish. The vessels appear smaller in size and the disc is clearly outlined.

Tabo-Paresis

Tabes and paresis may occur as intermediate or combined forms; for example, a tabetic onset followed by paretic mental changes, instead of ataxia. Thus it may be found that the C.S.F. of a clinically typical tabes shows the pattern seen in general paralysis of the insane. Such cases, if untreated, later show mental changes.

Syphilis of the Peripheral Nerves

This may arise when they are implicated in the syphilitic processes affecting the neighbouring structures, for example infiltrations of the nerve sheath, with irregular or cone-shaped thickenings; or from a gumma or lepto-meningitis, involving the anterior or posterior roots of the spinal cord, with characteristic sequelae of compression.

Neuralgia can occur without apparent anatomical basis. The facial nerve, the intercostals and the branches of the cervical or brachial plexus are most frequently involved. Severe pain is complained of and tender spots occur along the course of the affected nerve. Specific treatment effects rapid improvement.

Asymptomatic Neurosyphilis

This may be present in any case of late syphilis; that is, especially in syphilis of more than two to three years' duration. The cerebrospinal fluid must be examined in order to make the diagnosis or to exclude it. and to distinguish the condition from a late latent syphilis (p. 183).

Examination of the Cerebrospinal Fluid

For confirmation of the diagnosis or exclusion of neurosyphilis, and in the control of treatment, examination of the cerebrospinal fluid (C.S.F.) is of the utmost importance. It should be carried out in *all* cases of active late syphilis, whether there are signs present of central nervous system damage or not. All cases of treated early syphilis should have C.S.F. examination before they are discharged, if the response to treatment has not been completely satisfactory. The specimen of cerebrospinal fluid is usually obtained by a lumbar puncture. Cisternal puncture is not advocated for general use.

Lumbar Puncture

The specimen of cerebrospinal fluid is obtained by the introduction of a needle between the third and fourth, or fourth and fifth spinous processes of the lumbar vertebrae after entering the subarachnoid space. No special equipment is needed apart from a lumbar puncture needle of, for example, the Harris or the Dattner pattern. The technique is well-known; the operation may be carried out with the patient sitting up or lying down (p. 193).

Changes in the Cerebrospinal Fluid in Neurosyphilis

In neurosyphilis the macroscopic appearances of the C.S.F. are unaltered. In syphilitic meningitis and the early stages of general paralysis of the insane, cell counts of over 250 per c.mm. may be met with. A moderate increase of from 10 (above the upper limit of normal) to 50 cells per c.mm. is more usual, and is found in all forms of neurosyphilis. Small lymphocytes predominate; plasma cells may, however, be present.

The total protein and globulin content of the spinal fluid is consistently increased in all types of neurosyphilis, a very marked excess being common in syphilitic paresis and tabes; the upper limit of normal fluid usually is 45 mgs per 100 ml. with no increase in globulin.

A positive C.S.F. antibody reaction (Wassermann) is proof of neurosyphilis. However, a negative Wassermann reaction or equivalent test does not necessarily exclude syphilis of the central nervous system; the reaction may be negative in some cases of tabes dorsalis, cerebral gumma, and syphilitic disease of the cerebral vessels. A negative Wassermann in the C.S.F. in the presence of general paresis should make one reconsider the diagnosis.

The gold-sol or similar test is of value in differentiating between the various types of neurosyphilis, a positive response being elicited in the majority of cases. However, the reaction is not peculiar to syphilis, and other diseases, for example disseminated sclerosis or meningeal inflammation, may produce midzone or late zone changes. Whereas syphilitic paresis characteristically present with changes in the first part of the curve, in tabes dorsalis there is likely to be a midzone change giving a hump-back curve.

TREATMENT OF NEUROSYPHILIS

Neurosyphilis in its *acute* phase responds promptly to antibiotic therapy. Thus in the majority of cases, when there is active disease, a complete recovery follows treatment: an initial course of procaine penicillin therapy, 1·0 mega-unit, daily (or twice daily in the in-patient) by intramuscular injection for three weeks, followed by further courses of treatment. It is usual to choose a preparation of procaine penicillin but benzathine penicillin is as effective. For an acute illness or in cases responding sluggishly, the injections may be fortified with 1·0 mega-unit of watery benzyl penicillin given twice daily. It has to be remembered that treponemes have been isolated from the C.S.F. of treated neurosyphilis (p. 11). *Herxheimer reactions* may be expected in some cases, especially where there is more active disease, and precautions should be taken (p. 69).

If the patient is sensitive to penicillin, tetracycline should be used. The effect of its action is, in the main, less satisfactory than penicillin. Moderately high doses have to be used (0·5–1·0 g. six-hourly by mouth for two or three weeks), and the patient should then be kept under careful observation.

The serum antibody tests should show a slow decline in titre, and the C.S.F. become normal in about six months. Since treponemes have been isolated from the C.S.F. in treated neurosyphilis, retreatment is especially advisable in cases of neurosyphilis.

General care of health, diet, personal worries, living conditions, with rest in the early stages, are important. *Special care* must be given to the individual types of disorder. Other methods of attacking the treponeme in the central nervous system, used in the past in paresis, have no place in the treatment of this condition. The case of paresis often requires psychiatric attention, and social rehabilitation may be necessary before returning home or to a job: it is better to send such a patient to their previous environment rather than to an altered one.

Symptomatic treatment should be undertaken whenever the need arises. In the tabetic patient *pains* may respond to specific therapy. If not, simple analgesic drugs may be tried, for example, aspirin, phenacetin, paracetamol (0·5 g.); in resistant cases it might be necessary to use stronger drugs such as pethidine (25 mg.), physeptone (5–10 mg.) or morphine (10–20 mg. by injection), which are frequently necessary in *visceral crises*, for short periods. Corticosteroid therapy can be tried (p. 164).

Tabetic patients may benefit from short courses of vitamin supplements, or a course of vitamin B_{12} (1 million units injected daily). Patients with urinary *incontinence*, *ataxia*, *perforating ulcer* of the foot, or *Charcot's disease* of the joints require special measures since, having arisen and having failed to respond to specific treatment, these complications tend to persist.

Optic atrophy will not respond to special treatment, although the effect of steroid therapy together with antibiotics may be tried with some success in early cases. The prognosis in severe cases is poor (p. 77).

Late Latent Syphilis

Asymptomatic or latent syphilis is commoner in women than in men. Experimentally it can be shown that in the rabbit, oestrogen drugs protect the male animal from the more damaging results of infection with the treponeme.

Although latent late syphilis causes no obvious ill-health, it is known that the life-expectancy of such individuals is shortened by a number of years (from life-tables, about 10 per cent). In the younger patients there is always the danger that a damaging visceral complication will arise.

Treatment appears to protect the patient against any further manifestations of late syphilis, and a course of at least 10 mega-units of procaine penicillin should be given. A period for observation of the response in the serological titres is necessary.

A pregnant woman with untreated late latent syphilis may infect her foetus throughout her fertile period of life.

TREATMENT

See section on treatment of cardiovascular syphilis (p. 67).

CHAPTER 5

Congenital Syphilis

INTRODUCTION

'Congenital' syphilis is an infection of the foetus *via* the placental capillaries. The infection therefore does not occur until about the twelfth week of pregnancy. A spirochaetaemia in the mother is of variable occurrence, and the infection shows itself haphazardly in the siblings, the severity on the whole declining with the number of pregnancies. The existence of the disease is due to failure to diagnose and treat all cases of *maternal syphilis.*

'Paternal' transmission (*i.e.* infection of the foetus from infected semen without infection of the mother) does not occur. In syphilis acquired late in pregnancy, for example after the eighth month, the infant may escape intra-uterine infection, but develop a sore after the usual incubation period; the infection in such a case having occurred during birth.

The sequelae of congenital syphilis are similar to those of syphilis acquired by other routes, the main difference being that there is no primary sore. The disease may interfere with normal growth and lead to well-marked stigmata. Signs of congenital syphilis do not always occur soon after birth; signs are frequently delayed until the age of 15–20 years. Some can reach adult years without signs of ill-health.

The manifestations of congenital syphilis occurring under 2 years of age may be considered as *early*, and those at any later age as *late*. The early congenital syphilis corresponds in many respects with those of early 'acquired' syphilis. Late congenital syphilis, although exhibiting many manifestations similar to those of late 'acquired' syphilis, shows, in addition, various stigmata, scars of developmental abnormalities resulting from previously active syphilitic lesions. A truly asymptomatic infection may also occur; no symptoms, signs or stigmata being present until the appearance of later clinical manifestations. A syphilitic infant cannot infect its own mother (Colles), and a mother with manifest syphilis can suckle her own apparently normal infant without infecting it (Profeta). Clinical manifestations of congenital syphilis are *uncommon within three or four weeks of birth*; the earlier clinical signs appear, the more severe the infection. Late manifestations of congenital syphilis vary greatly in the time of appearance, but not uncommonly occur between the ages of five and seven years, at puberty, or about the twentieth year.

The most severely infected are still-born.

Early Congenital Syphilis

The serological tests for antibodies in the young infant's serum will be for maternal antibodies for a time, due to passive-transfer before birth. In order that these tests should truly demonstrate the infant's antibodies, they are best performed on the infant's serum not earlier than six weeks after birth. Before this time, active infection in the infant has to be judged on clinical grounds.

The infection varies greatly. Those who are severely infected are often irritable, suffering from fits of crying, disturbed sleep and bouts of pyrexia. Wasting may be present together with a wrinkled, 'cafe au lait' and 'wizened' facies.

Skin

Papulo-squamous eruptions, like those of early acquired infection, are usual in severe cases and affect the buttocks, 'nappy area', palms, soles, and naso-labial region. Bullous eruptions may occur on the legs, palms, soles, forearm and face: so-called 'syphilitic pemphigus'. Diagnosis from other dermatological conditions has been discussed. The 'nappy rash' is pink and irritative, and is accompanied by a typical ammoniacal smell. Wasting disorder and failure to thrive in infancy, where the mother's serum has not been tested, should indicate the need for such a serum test to exclude syphilis: this will always be positive in an infected infant.

Mucosal Lesions

These correspond with those in early infectious 'acquired syphilis'. The infant suffers from '*snuffles*' due to mucosal

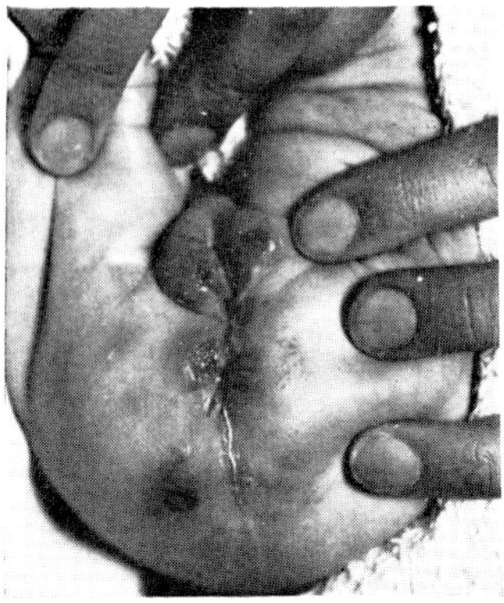

FIG. 90.

Vulval and anal moist patches in the infant.

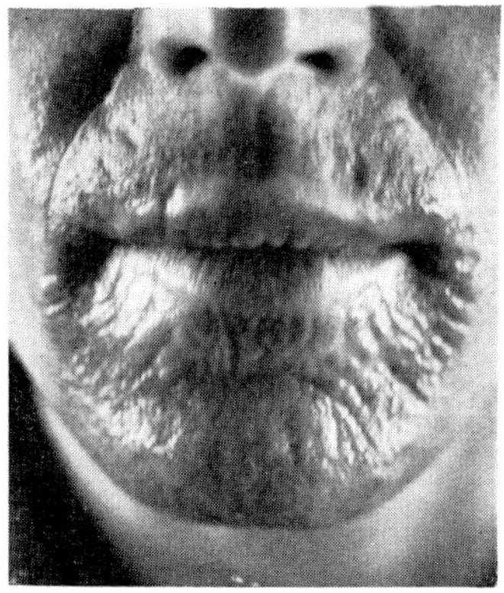

FIG. 91.

Rhagades in the young adult.

eruptions, causing slight obstruction to breathing and difficulty in suckling. '*Saddle-nose*' results from spread of the lesions causing erosion of cartilage and bony necrosis. *Laryngitis* occurs. '*Rhagades*', or scarring, resulting from fissures about the mouth, are pathognomonic but do not always occur. Patchy thinning of the *hair* may be preceded by excessive growth ('syphilitic mop'). Lymphadenitis is common, as is visceral enlargement.

PERIOSTITIS, OSTEITIS AND OSTEOCHONDRITIS

These conditions may exist almost from birth, or develop later. Osteitis is rare in congenital syphilis: periostitis of the long bones is commoner. Lesions of the *epiphyses* may be noted on X-ray examination in the early weeks of life, and are usually accompanied by marked tnederness, swelling and loss of use of the limb. X-ray of the epiphysis shows a broadened, irregular, wavy and opaque band. The condition is readily distinguished from scurvy, ricketts, and infant myxoedema. Thinning of the occipital and parietal bones occurs (as in ricketts), 'craniotabes'; or

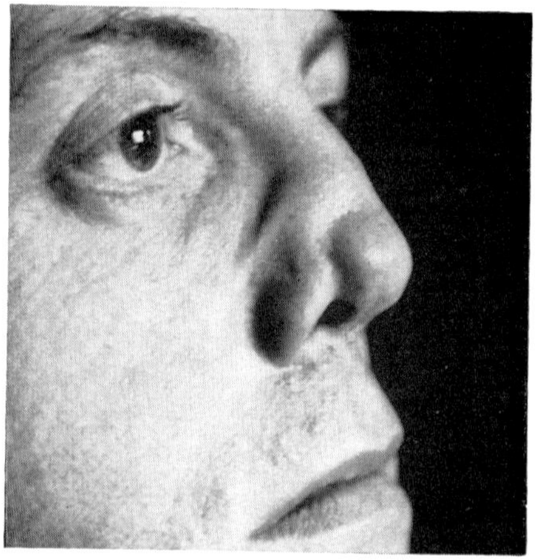

FIG. 92.

Osteitis and chondritis of nasal bone and cartilage in late congenital syphilis.

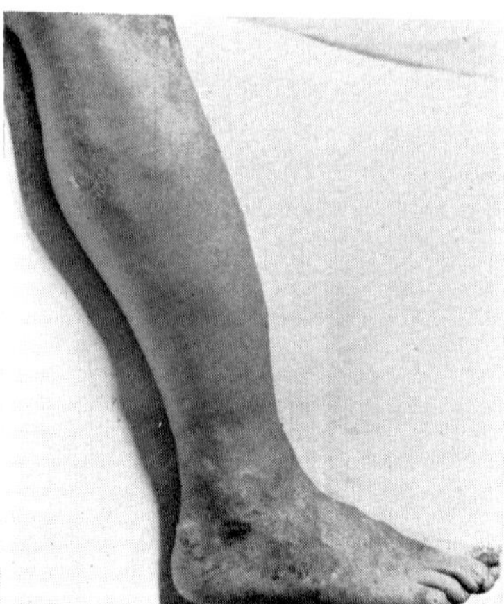

FIG. 93.

'Sabre-shin' tibia.

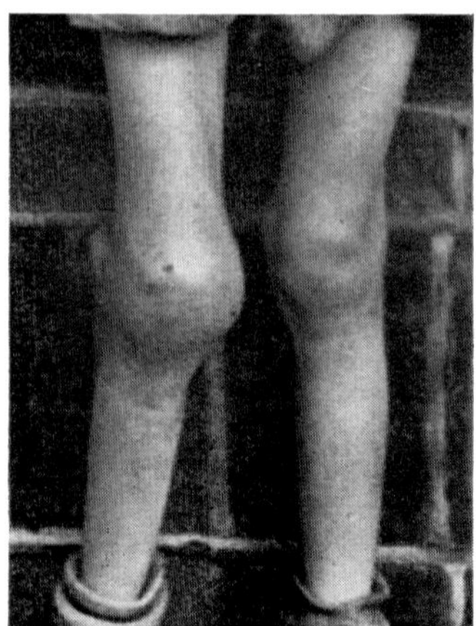

FIG. 94.

Neglected Clutton's Joint—commencing osteochondro-arthritis.

thickening of the frontal and parietal bones about the anterior fontanelle, resulting in a square or naciform 'Parrot's nodes' or 'hot cross bun' skull.

Lesions of the viscera and central nervous system in infancy are rare. However such lesions as *hydrocephalus*, or basal *meningitis*, may arise in the first year of life. Enlargement of the *spleen* and *liver* is not uncommon; the liver being smooth, firm and tender. The condition responds well to treatment. Albuminuria can occur. Iritis, optic neuritis and disseminated *choroiditis* may be noted; the latter of the larger patchy kind or of the spidery variety (to be distinguished from retinitis pigmentosa).

'*White pneumonia*' is met with in still-born infants or those surviving but a few days. There is marked interstitial fibrosis with characteristic cellular changes.

Late Congenital Syphilis

A great diversity is to be found in the late manifestations of congenital syphilis. The signs of this disorder fall into two groups: *stigmata*, the results of early active infection; and signs of active *progressive lesions*. The serological tests are invariably positive; although later in life certain of the tests tend to become negative. Particularly after adolescence the presence of stigmata are of great importance in the clinical diagnosis of congenital syphilis, suggesting the presence of what today is a rare disease. When congenital syphilis is suspected it is useful to test the serum of the mother and other members of the family.

OSTEOPERIOSTITIS

This is seen at about 8 years of age. The tibiae are more commonly affected than other parts, the sclerosing process resulting in a thickening with 'sabre shin' deformity. The commonest joint lesion is a painless *hydrarthrosis* involving one or both knees (Clutton's joints). It occurs in early adolescence, having an insidious onset, and is due to a gummatous synovitis. There is no abnormality in the X-ray. Spontaneous recovery with no deformity occurs even in the untreated.

EYES, EARS AND TEETH

Lesions of the eye are frequent in congenital syphilis. *Iritis* occurs at any time after birth and is often associated with choroiditis. *Optic atrophy* may occur alone or accompanying involvement of the central nervous system.

Interstitial keratitis is frequent after the seventh year, one, and subsequently both eyes being involved. The lesion appears in over 50 per cent of the cases and is typical of congenital syphilis. It is due to interference by the disease in the foetal development of the cornea. The lesion begins insidiously, with photophobia and the presence of ciliary injection, followed by a patchy opalescence of the central cornea. 'Pink patches' form in the cornea, due to the presence of capillaries, which are followed eventually by scarring and varying degrees of loss of vision. Several attacks may occur, leading in the untreated case to near-blindness, Specific therapy does not completely protect the patient against relapse, which occurs with such precipitating factors as trauma, pregnancy or ill-health. Corticosteroids should

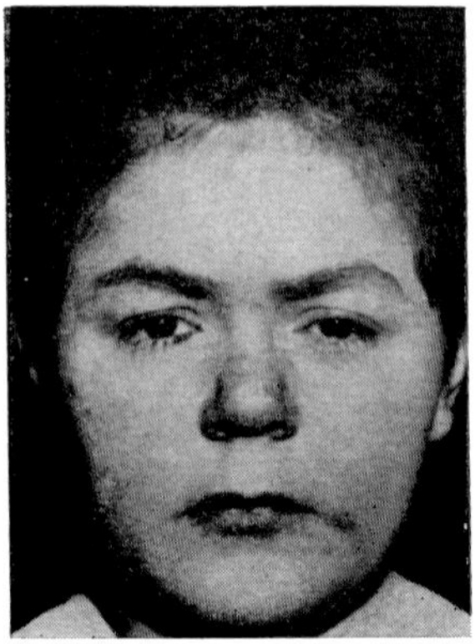

FIG. 95.

Photophobia of keratitis and 'platter facies'.

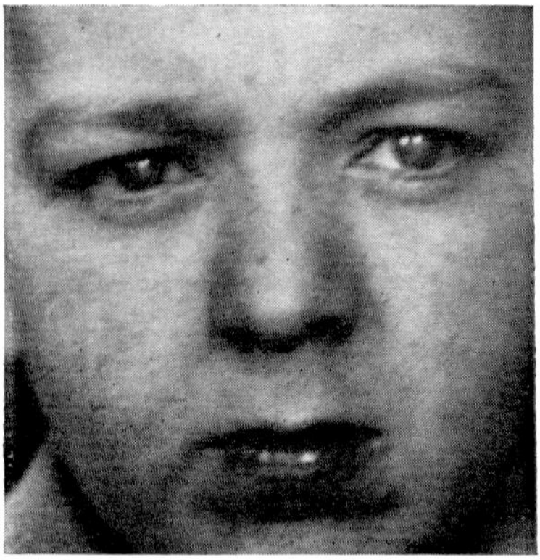

FIG. 96.

Interstitial keratitis, showing corneal opacity and down-drawn eyebrows of photophobic habitus.

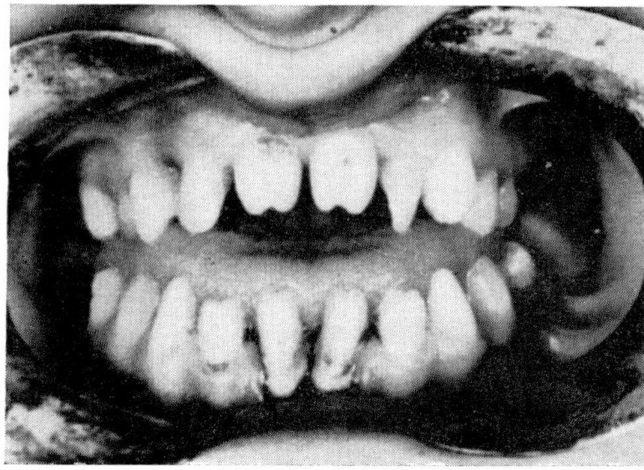

FIG. 97.
Hutchinson's Teeth.

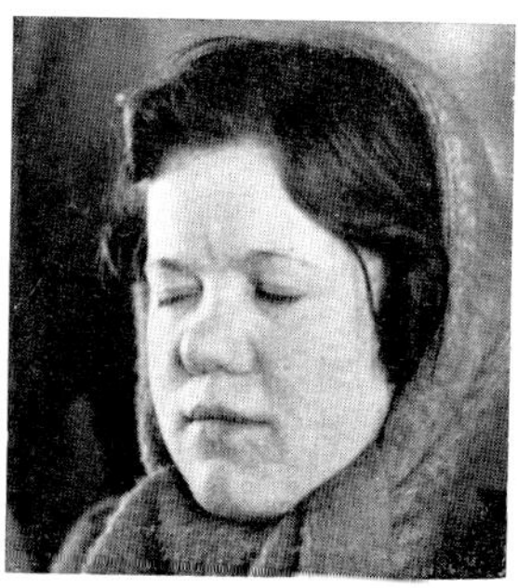

FIG. 98.
'Dish-shaped' facies of congenital syphilis.

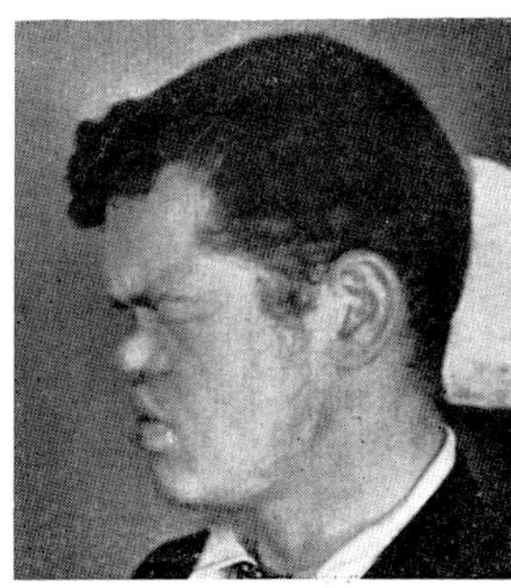

FIG. 99.
Typical facies of congenital syphilis.

be applied locally in the form of an ointment or eye-drops, *i.e.* Predsol or Betnesol 0·5 or 1 per cent.

A suppurative *otitis media* is rarely met with in the early case.

Eighth cranial *nerve deafness* can occur from the age of 7 years onwards, the triad of keratitis, deafness and dental stigmata being known as *Hutchinson's triad.*

Deformities of the *permanent dentition* occur in congenital syphilis and are due to interference by the disease in the developing structures. There is a defect of dentine and enamel; the incisor teeth are wedge- or peg-shaped with knotched cutting edges, and are widely spaced (Hutchinson's teeth). The lower incisors are much less affected. Similarly the first permanent molars, especially the lower, are affected, giving rise to rounded cusps. All such teeth rapidly suffer from caries.

The typical *facies* of late congenital syphilis is now seldom met with. Rhagades, corneal haze, flattened nasal bridge with frontal bossing is unmistakable when it occurs. A so-called 'dish-facies' is more common, due to underdevelopment of the pre-maxilla, the face tending to be concave both from forehead to chin, and transversely.

NEUROSYPHILIS

It is now recognised that in prenatal syphilis involvement of the central nervous system is less infrequent than was formerly believed. The symptoms, signs and clinical findings may be little marked, and the condition progresses insidiously unless detected by careful examination. The basal *meningitis* of early congenital syphilis may be asymptomatic, or it may be associated with irritability, convulsions and cranial nerve paralyses, be followed by hydrocephalus, and later by the occurrence of epilepsy and mental deficiency. Cerebrovascular lesions occur at any time. Parenchymatous neurosyphilis becomes manifest about the age of puberty, but can be delayed to the age of 25: in juvenile paresis the individual, who previously was mentally normal, shows progressive mental deterioration, becoming backward and careless at school or at work. Emotional instability is shown by sudden fits of temper, night terrors, perversity, the development of an unruly wildness or outright delinquency. Epileptiform fits may be an early sign. Delusions or mental exaltation seldom occur.

Juvenile tabes is frequently asymptomatic and can be detected only by careful examination.

Cardiovascular disorder occurs very rarely in congenital syphilis.

Treatment of Congenital Syphilis

The treatment should begin as soon as the diagnosis is confirmed. The effect of *penicillin* therapy in early congenital syphilis is comparable to its action in acquired syphilis, causing rapid healing of the muco-cutaneous and osseous lesions, and diminution of the serological titre. Children tolerate large dosages and, for infants treated shortly after birth, a total of 0·5 mega-unit per kg. body weight of procaine penicillin is given intramuscularly, in divided dosage, over 12 days. With aqueous benzyl penicillin, four-hourly administration should be employed. Oral penicillin is not so effective, but may have to be resorted to where there is insufficient muscle for daily injections. (250 mg. phenethicillin as crushed tablet or syrup is given six-hourly for two weeks.) In rare cases, for example of marasmus or gross visceral lesions, in which the consequences of a Herxheimer reaction might prove serious, prior treatment with iodides (potassium iodide 0·25–0·5 g. daily for a few days) or prednisolone 5 mg. should be considered. In most instances it is wise to start antibiotic treatment as soon as possible.

The treatment of congenital syphilis at later periods in life is carried out on lines comparable to those in adult-acquired syphilis; the sole modifications being the employment of doses suitable to the age, weight and condition of the patient, and the necessary protraction of treatment in sero-resistant cases. Where the patient is sensitised to penicillin, *tetracycline* should be used, 20 mg./kg. weight daily (p. 210), in divided dosage for two weeks. In congenital syphilis the *serological tests* have a tendency to remain positive, sometimes in moderately high titre, despite treatment. Only observation will show whether the disease is satisfactorily treated and the patient healthy in such circumstances. However, when the patient reaches adulthood, the disease usually remains quiescent, with the exception of the lesion of keratitis.

Interstitial keratitis, due to congenital syphilis, is treated with local corticosteroid (prednisolone oculentum 1 per cent); and disorders of the middle ear with systemic corticosteroid (prednisolone 5·0 mg. daily, to be tailed off; as a rule, two to three weeks' treatment).

These corticosteroid drugs are given along with antibiotic therapy, and they are used during the active phase of the particular attack. Occasionally such treatment has to be prolonged; but there are dangers to the use of corticosteroids in infants, since these drugs affect growth.

MATERNAL SYPHILIS
(Syphilis in Pregnancy)

Pregnancy has little adverse effect on the course of acquired syphilis. There is often, indeed, a marked tendency to mitigation of the disease. The primary sore is trivial and involutes rapidly, the secondary manifestations are entirely absent and unaccompanied by constitutional symptoms. The effect of syphilis on child-bearing depends on the time of infection; syphilis may have been acquired at some time prior to conception, at the time of conception, or at some later period during pregnancy. Depending upon the duration of the infection, the sequence of early miscarriage or still-births, living syphilitic children or healthy children may result. It is assumed that during the course of an untreated syphilis there are recurrent waves of spirochaetaemia, varying in frequency and duration according to the age of the infection, and it is during one of these periods that the foetus may become infected. This explains the greater risk of foetal infection in early syphilis and the later vagaries of transmission of syphilis from an infected mother to her offspring. Where there has been a large number of pregnancies the typical pattern in syphilis is that of live births interspersed with miscarriages or deaths in infancy, the overall picture improving with the number of pregnancies. The serum tests are usually positive.

Third generation syphilis, or the transmission of infection from an untreated 'congenital syphilitic' mother to her foetus, is by no means unknown.

The typical *syphilitic placenta* is larger than normal and its weight ratio to that of the foetus is one to four as compared with the normal one to six. It is pale and 'greasy looking'; its consistency is softer and sometimes almost friable. Infarcts are numerous. Microscopically, characteristic vascular and perivascular changes are seen, the chorionic villi are thicker and more club-shaped, and the stroma cells are closely packed instead of being stellate. An apparently normal placenta may be found despite the foetus being undoubtedly syphilitic.

The institution of treatment for syphilis at the earliest possible moment in pregnancy is of the utmost importance if a healthy child is to be secured. The serum tests for syphilis should be performed as a routine on every expectant mother, since the history is often of little help in these cases. The problem of the non-syphilitic positive serum Wassermann reaction has already been discussed (p. 46).

TREATMENT OF SYPHILIS DURING PREGNANCY

This should eliminate 'congenital' syphilis. The effectiveness of penicillin in protecting the foetus from maternal syphilis, even if treatment is delayed until as late as the last two months of pregnancy, is widely recognised. The usual course of treatment is for procaine penicillin to be injected intramuscularly, 1 million units daily for 10 days or two weeks. If the titre of the quantitative test remains high and shows no decline after three months, re-treatment is indicated. It is no longer considered necessary to re-treat, during each and every subsequent pregnancy, women with borderline tests who have already had adequate treatment for their syphilis. But in certain cases, for example where there is a high serological titre or clinical disease, courses of re-treatment with penicillin are advised.

ENDEMIC SYPHILIS

This condition may be seen in primitive communities. If the disease is so common in the infective stage as to be transferred non-venereally by young children, it is not often transmitted *via* the placenta (congenital disease) since women in the childbearing years have already reached the late, more quiescent, stages of the disease.

The communal 'one-shot' treatment with a repository penicillin (2–3 mega-units benzathine penicillin) is thought to eliminate the disease in this form. Daily treatment is preferable.

SELECTED BIBLIOGRAPHY FOR SYPHILIS

General and Historical

WORLD FORUM ON SYPHILIS
Publ. Hlth Serv. Publs. Wash. (1964). No. 997
RISE AND FALL OF THE TREPONEMATOSES
Idsoe, O. & Guthe, T. (1967). *Br. J. vener. Dis.* **43,** 227.
Idsoe, O. & Guthe, T. (1968). *Br. J. vener. Dis.* **44,** 35.
SYPHILIS MALIGNA PRAECOX
Cripps, D. J. & Curtis, A. C. (1967). *Archs intern. Med.* **119,** 411.
SYPHILIS PAST AND PRESENT
Lancet, (1967). **2,** 503.

Immune Aspects and Biology of the Organism

IMMUNITY IN EXPERIMENTAL SYPHILIS
Miller, J. N. (1967). *J. Immunol.* **99,** 1012.
IMMUNITY IN SYPHILIS
Cannefax, G. R., Norris, L. C. & Gillespie, E. J. (1967). *Am. Rev. Med.* **18,** 471.
Wigfield, A. S. (1965). *Br. J. vener. Dis.* **41,** 275.
ELECTRONMICROSCOPIC STUDIES OF THE TREPONEMA PALLIDUM
Oveinnikov, N. M. & Delectorskij, W. (1968). *Br. J. vener. Dis.* **43** 227; **44,** 35.
T. PALLIDUM: BIBLIOGRAPHICAL REVIEW
Willcox, R. R. & Guthe, T. (1966). *Bull. Wld Hlth Org.* No. 35.
REITER TREPONEME
Wallace, A. L. & Mans, A. (1967). *Bull. Wld Hlth Org.* No. 36.
BIOLOGY OF THE TREPONEMATOSES
Turner, T. B. & Hollander, D. H. (1957). *Monograph Ser. Wld Hlth Org.* No. 35.

Clinical:

FLUORESCENT AND CONVENTIONAL DARK-FIELD METHODS OF DIAGNOSIS
Jue, R., Puffer, J. Wood, R. M., Schochet, G., Smartt, W. H. & Ketterer, W. A. (1967). *Am. J. clin. Path.* **47,** 809.

RE-INFECTION (45 CASES)

Burgess, A., Salvador, R., Dupre, A., Parant, M. & Christol, B. (1966). *Proph. saint. morale*, **38,** 107.

LATE SYPHILIS; REVIEW OF RECENT LITERATURE

Nicholas, L. & Barrman, H. (1967). *Am. J. med. Sci.*, **254,** 549.

TREATMENT OF EARLY SYPHILIS

Mach, K. (1967). *Wien klin. Wschr.* **79,** 97.

TREATMENT OF SYPHILIS

King, A. J. (1965). *Practitioner*, **195,** 589.

SERODIAGNOSIS AND TREATMENT OF SYPHILIS

Olansky, S. & Norris, L. C. (1966). *J. Am. med. Ass.* **198,** 165.

SERONEGATIVE MATERNAL SYPHILIS

Tinkler, A. E. (1968). *Br. J. vener. Dis.* **44,** 136.

TREATMENT FAILURE (EXAMPLE—NEUROSYPHILIS OCCURRING WITHIN YEAR OF THERAPY)

Hewitt, A. B. (1967). *Br. J. vener. Dis.* **43,** 272.

TREPONEMES ISOLATED FROM TREATED SYPHILIS

Smith, J. Lawton & Israel, C. W. (1968). *Br. J. vener. Dis.* **44,** 109.

Yobs, A. R., Clark, J. W., Mothershed, S. E., Bullard, J. C. & Artley, C. W. (1968). *Br. J. vener. Dis.* **44,** 116.

Serological

COMPARISON FTA-ABS WITH TPI TEST ON OVER 1000 PROBLEM SERA

Johnston, N. A. & Wilkinson, A. E. (1968). *Br. J. vener. Dis.* **44,** [In press.]

Wood, R. M., Mouye, Y., Argouza, W., Bradford, L., Jue, R., Jeong, Y., Puffer, J. & Bodily, H. L. (1967). *Am. J. clin. Path.* **47,** 521.

MODERN SERO-DIAGNOSIS OF SYPHILIS

Muller, F. (1967). *Münch. med. Wschr.* **109,** 1591.

REITER PROTEIN COMPLEMENT FIXATION TEST

see Reiter treponeme loc. cit.

BIOLOGICAL FALSE POSITIVE REACTIONS: IMMUNO-ELECTROPHORESIS

Kiraly, K. Keldor, Jobbagy, A., & Karsai K. (1966). *Acta dermato.-vener. Stockh.* **46,** 506.

BIOLOGICAL FALSE POSITIVE REACTIONS: INCIDENCE IN PREGNANCY

Lee, K. (1966). *Tidsskh. norske Laegforen.* **86,** 1728.

CHAPTER 6

Chancroid; Granuloma Inguinale; Lymphogranuloma Venereum

These three conditions are transmitted venereally in a large proportion of cases. They have usually been described together since they are causes of genital 'sores'; they are moreover relatively rare, and tend to be limited to warmer climates or sea-board cities.

CHANCROID (Soft Chancre, Soft Sore)

Chancroid is a localised painful genital ulceration, due to a Gram-negative bacillus, *Haemophilus ducreyi*. The incubation period is short, three to five days. The disease is subject to local complications: lymphangitis, bubo formation and phagedena, but never causes a constitutional illness. Extragenital chancroids rarely occur; contagion from infected linen, and auto-inoculation, for example of the fingers from the genital lesions, is possible. Men, especially among the less hygienic individuals, and itinerants such as seamen, are more frequently affected than women. Examination of the alleged sources of infection may reveal no recognisable chancroidal lesions in the female, suggesting the possibility of asymptomatic infectivity or 'carrier' state.

The common sites of infection are: in men, the coronal sulcus, frenum, preputial meatus, urethral meatus, or glans penis; and in women the vulva, perineum, labia majora and minora, urethra, thighs, vagina or cervix, in order of frequency. The disease progresses rapidly from a vesico-pustule to a sharply circumscribed ragged ulcer with undetermined edges, presenting varied degrees of severity. The base of the ulcer is covered with a greyish exudate. An erythematous areola surrounds the lesion, which is markedly tender and painful. Auto-inoculation results in multiple lesions. Bubo formation sometimes occurs and may progress to suppuration, rupture and ragged ulceration.

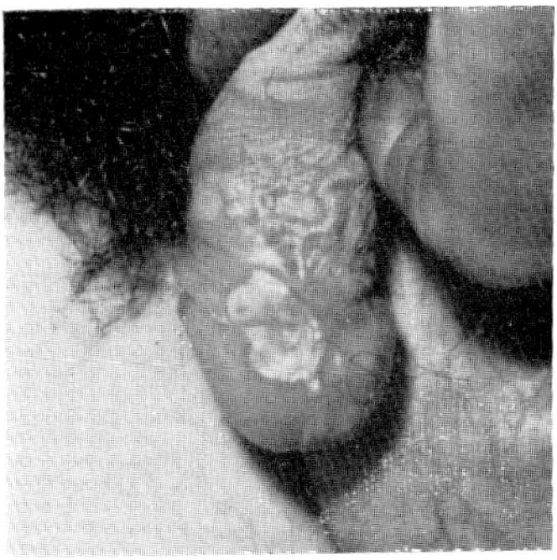

FIG. 100.

Ulcer in region of frenum due to chancroid.

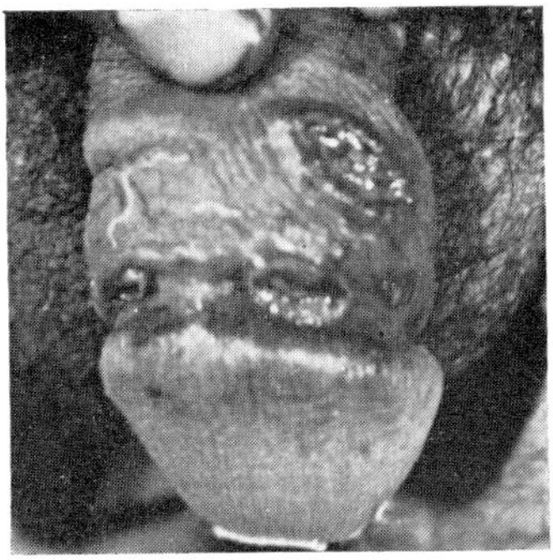

FIG. 101.

Multiple chancroidal ulcers on coronal sulcus and inner aspect of prepuce.

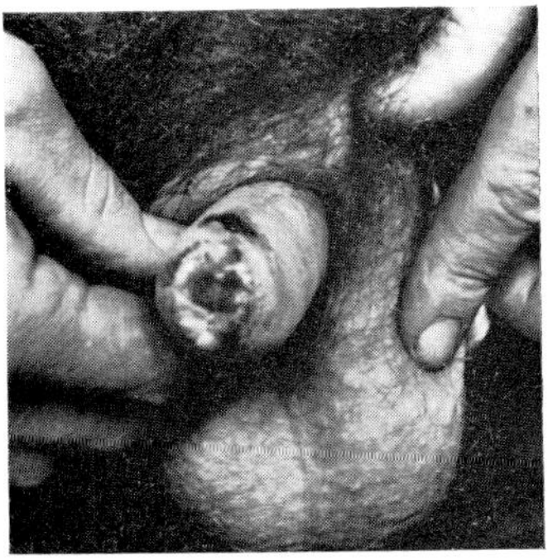

FIG. 102.

Chancroid of corona glandis, and fluctuating bubo.

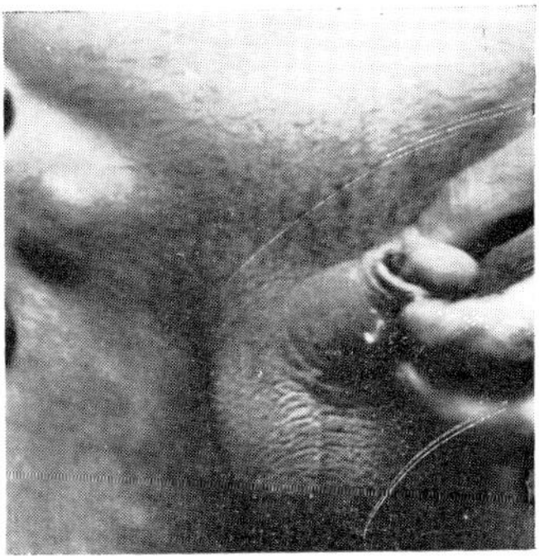

FIG. 103.

Chancroidal ulceration of preputial meatus, showing typical 'fuzzy' appearance.

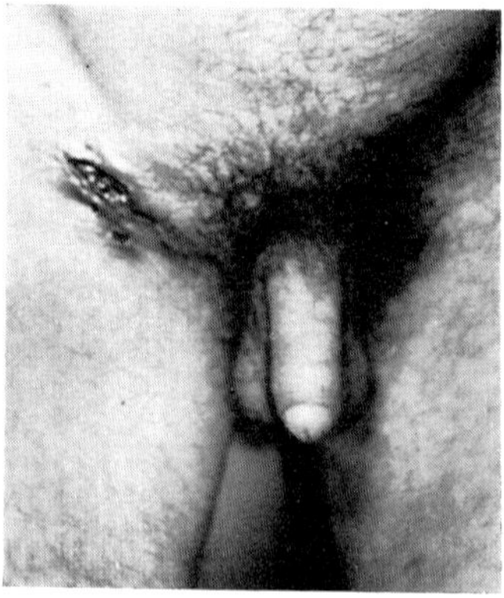

FIG. 104.

Groin ulceration following rupture of bubo.

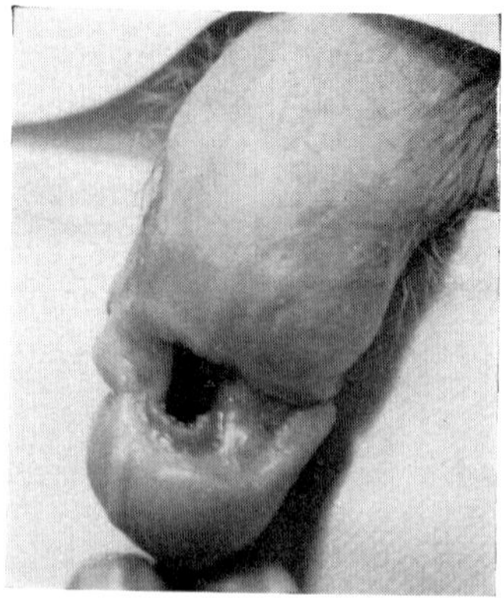

FIG. 105.

Urethral fistula following chancroidal ulceration of frenal area.

DIAGNOSIS

This is confirmed by recovering the 'ducrey' bacillus from the edges of the lesions, and staining a smear preparation with Gram stain. *B. ducreyi* is a small, slender Gram-negative bacillus, more heavily staining at either end. Culture of the organism is not easy.

TREATMENT

In the first instance, treatment should be with sulphonamides until *syphilis* has been excluded: a long-acting sulphonamide 1·0 g. daily, or, for example, sulphatriad 1·0 g. four-hourly for 48 hours. Streptomycin 1·0 g. o.d. by intramuscular injection for five days may also be used. Bubos should be aspirated, never incised. For those cases which do not respond completely a course of tetracycline 5·0 g. by mouth in divided dosage may be given, after rigorous exclusion of syphilis.

GRANULOMA INGUINALE

This is an uncommon, moderately contagious, almost chronic disease involving skin, subcutaneous tissue and lymphatics. It seems to be transmitted by coitus. Generalised spread is rare and only occurs in debilitated persons. It is caused by the Donovan body (*Donovania granulomatis*), a minute protozoon recoverable from the lesions. It is strictly parasitic for man. The disease is seen in the tropics and mainly in the negro race.

The incubation period is uncertain and may be on average four to six weeks. The early lesion is a papule, vesicle or nodule which erodes and becomes an ulcer with a red granular base. It may present as a red, smooth mass of granulation tissue on the prepuce or vulva. The margins of the lesions are well defined; the lesions bleed easily but are not painful. They show little tendency to heal, and spread by contiguity, the advancing border having a rolled edge. The ulcerative process may remain almost stationary for years. Scarring occurs to some extent. The inguinal swelling in this disease is a subcutaneous granuloma not an adenitis. Ultimately impairment of health takes place. Granulomatosis, or spread into the body viscera, is rare. Such widespread disease may result in cachexia and death.

DIAGNOSIS

This is confirmed by taking a tissue scraping from the lesion, making a smear on a slide and staining this with Wright's or Giemsa's stain. The coccal- or diplococcal-like organism, surrounded by a halo of encapsulation and lying within large round epithelial cells, is typical of this condition.

Differential diagnosis must include ulceration due to such conditions as furospirochaetosis (Vincent's) and blastomycosis, amongst others.

TREATMENT

If courses with suitable antibiotics, are repeated, treatment is usually effective. Tetracycline by mouth, 0·5 g. q.d.s. for two

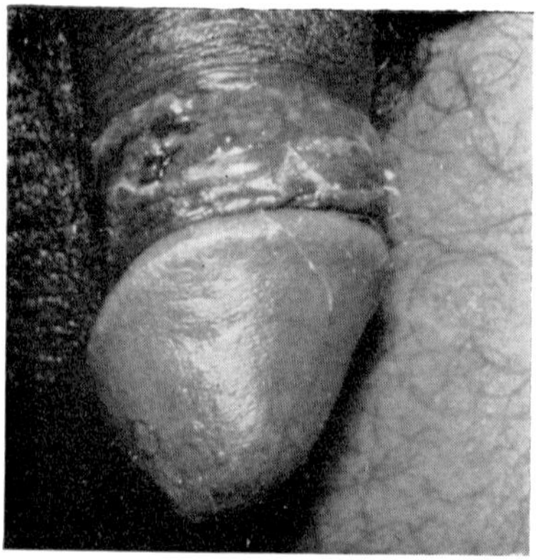

FIG. 106.
Granuloma inguinale of prepuce.

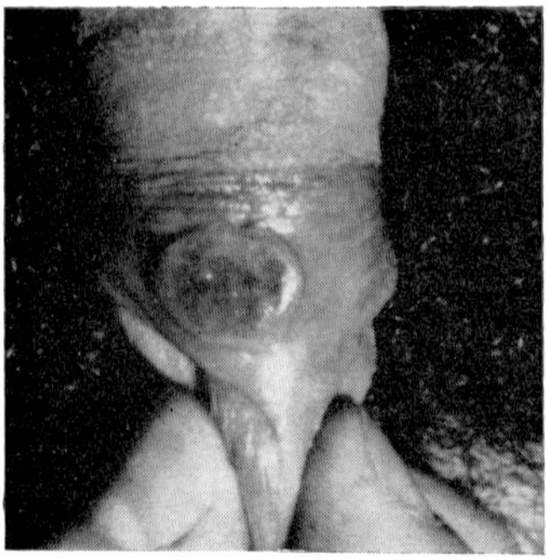

FIG. 107.
Granuloma inguinale.

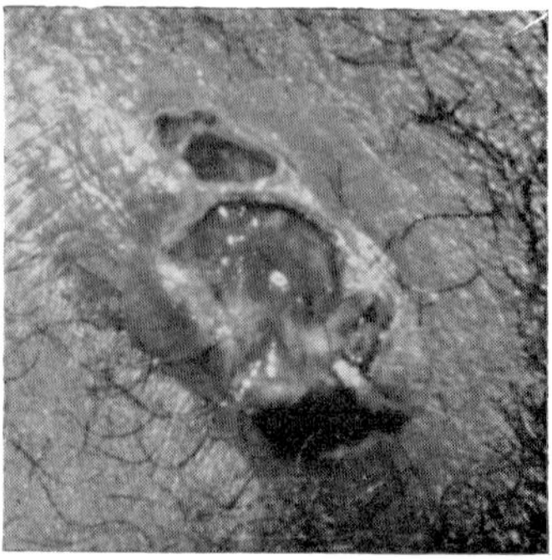

FIG. 108.
Granuloma inguinale of the inguinal region.

weeks; but streptomycin 1·0 g. o.d. by intramuscular injection for the same period, should be tried before syphilis has been excluded.

LYMPHOGRANULOMA VENEREUM

Lymphogranuloma venereum is due to the virus of the above name, and is acquired by coitus. It is widespread throughout the world, being seen more often in the warmer countries. To what extent the virus infects non-venereally (and outside laboratories) is not known. It spreads via the lymphatics and may result locally in bubo formation, ulceration, elephantiasis and rectal stricture. The disease is probably more common than is realised.

The incubation period is one to two weeks. A primary lesion is not always seen and consists of a minute papule or vesicle; but more often than not this is evanescent. The bubo is recognised up to a month later. A lesion on the penis results in inguinal adenitis, in the vagina a pelvi-rectal adenitis and in the ano-rectal region a perirectal adenitis. Occasionally the primary lesion heals, but chronic ulceration can occur locally.

The inguinal bubo (usually unilateral) is firm and elongated; the skin is adherent and has a discoloured hue. Irregular areas of softening develop, which is followed by suppuration and, ultimately, by the formation of fistulae.

Lymphatic blockage due to infection may result in genital elephantiasis (of the vulva, known as Esthiomene) and various pedunculated tumours of vulval tissue.

Vaginal or ano-rectal stricture can develop. Rectal stricture is also seen in the absence of any history or sign of primary lesion or bubo. The disease can be quite mild and the patient may never be aware of any infection. On the other hand it may manifest itself intermittently or more continuously over many years, resulting in pyrexia, debility or invalidism.

DIAGNOSIS

This is made by demonstrating skin hypersensitivity and confirming a positive result by means of a complement fixation test

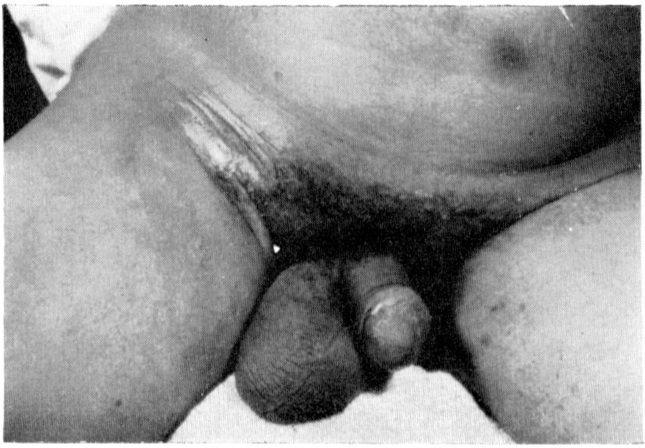

FIG. 109.

Lymphogranuloma venereum showing bubo of right groin and healing lesion near corona of glans.

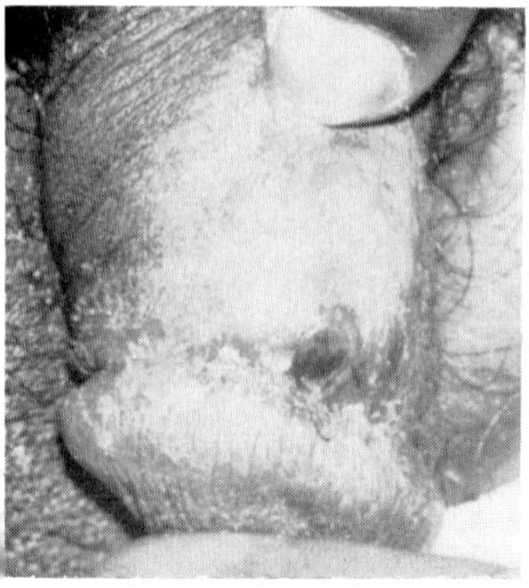

FIG. 110.

Ulcerated early lesion of lymphogranuloma venereum.

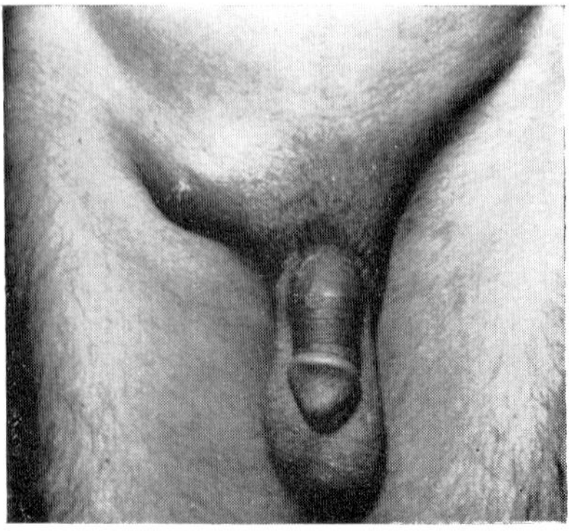

FIG. 111.

Bubo, early, of lymphogranuloma venereum.

on the patient's serum. In the 'skin test', 0·1 ml. Frei antigen, LGV virus, prepared in chick embryos, along with uninfected yolk-material as control, is injected intradermally in the forearm so that a wheal is raised. A papule, and erythema of at least 5 mm. diameter, is present at 48 hours in a positive case. More delayed reactions may occur. This must be followed by the complement fixation test in the patient's serum using LGV antigen.

Differential diagnosis should include any cause of an enlarged lymph node, local causes such as syphilis, chancroid, or other local infection such as tuberculosis or malignancy, or systemic disorders, for example Hodgkin's disease, and also less common conditions such as tularaemia, or causes of elephantic changes such as filariasis. Rectal inflammation, especially in women, must be excluded, such as neisserian infection, non-specific proctitis and regional enteritis.

TREATMENT

The disease responds slowly to large doses of sulphonamide or tetracycline. If the bubos become fluctulent they should be drained by aspiration, never by incision. In the event of rupture the ulcerated bubo is very slow to heal. Sulphatriad 1·0 g. four-hourly for 48 hours, followed by 1·0 g. six-hourly for four days is the treatment of choice before syphilis has been excluded. If syphilis is known to be absent, tetracycline is taken by mouth 0·5 g. six-hourly for five days and 0·25 g. six-hourly for a further nine days.

SELECTED BIBLIOGRAPHY

Chancroid

VDRL Chancroid Studies I, II & III
Olanski, S., Abritton, D. C., Kaplan, W. & Deacon, W. E. (1956). *J. invest. Derm.* **26**, 339, 407, 415.
Hyperimmune Reaction in Chancroid
Tyler, D. E. (1956). *U. S. arm. Forces med. J.* **7**, 663.

Granuloma Inguinale

Rajam, R. V. & Rangiah, P. N. (1954). 'Donovanasis'. *Monograph Ser. Wld Hlth Org*. No. 20.

Goldberg, J. & Annamunthodo, H. (1966). *J. vener. Dis.* **42,** 205.

CULTURE OF D. GRANULOMATIS

Lal S Singh, G. (1967). *Indian J. Derm. Vener.* **33,** 251.

Lymphogranuloma Venereum

Jorgensen, L. (1959). *Acta path. microbiol. scand.* **47,** 113.

REVIEW OF LITERATURE

World Health Organization (1954). *Vener. dis. trans.* p. 114.

PART 2

Gonorrhoea and Venereal Discharges

CHAPTER 7

Gonorrhoea

Gonorrhoea is a bacterial disease caused by the *Neisseria gonorrhoeae*, a 'Gram-negative diplococcus'. The primary site of infection is the non-keratinised epithelium and glands of the lower genito-urinary tract of men and women. Direct local extension of infection involves other genito-urinary structures, while blood-stream infection results in metastatic complications of which arthritis is the most common.

In almost all cases, genital infection with the 'gonococcus' follows *sexual* intercourse with an infected person. Accidental contagion of the male urethra is very rare indeed; non-sexual infection of the adult woman, for example from lavatory seats or infected towels, is theoretically possible. The majority of instances of such 'accidental' infection, however, are those of vulvo-vaginitis in girls before puberty, and neonatal and adult gonococcal ophthalmia, that is, purulent gonococcal conjunctivitis without concomitant genital infection. A knowledge of the anatomy of the genito-urinary tract in both sexes is essential if the possibilities of gonococcal infection are to be fully appreciated (Figs. 112–113).

In men, the interval between the time of implantation of the gonococcus on the urethral epithelium and the appearance of symptoms (incubation period), usually varies from four to seven days. The length of this incubation period depends on factors common to all infections: the virulence and dosage of the organism, the resistance of the infected person, and their ability to note symptoms. It seldom exceeds 14 days.

In women the symptoms of infection are frequently either trivial or, for other reasons, are disregarded. Most women therefore will not directly seek medical advice. It is of great importance to recognise this fact, and to persuade the male to approach his partner and suggest that she should be examined. A complete gynaecological and obstetric history should be taken in every case.

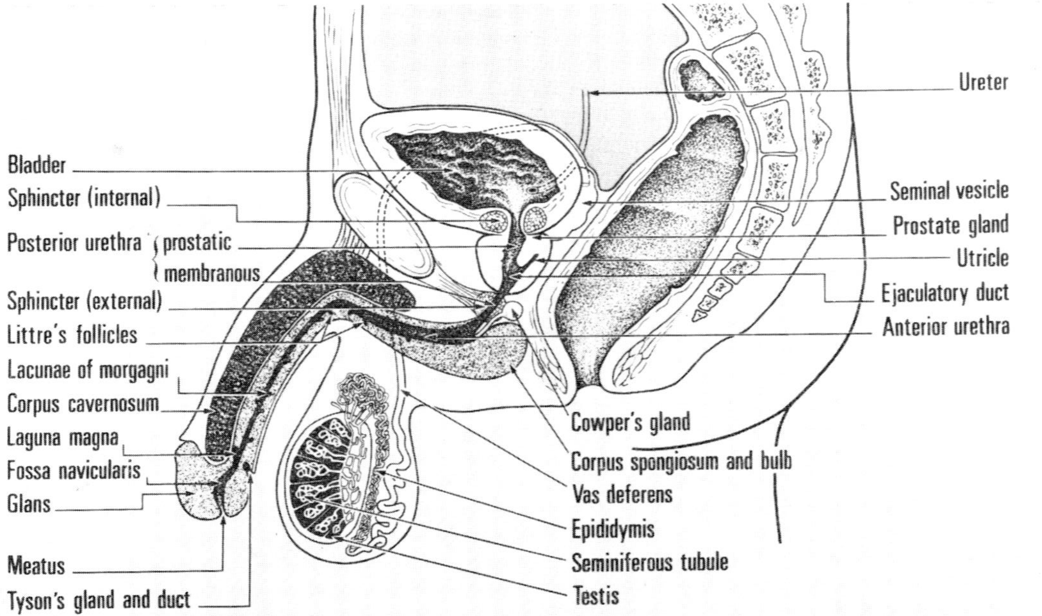

FIG. 112—Anatomical diagram of male genito-urinary tract.

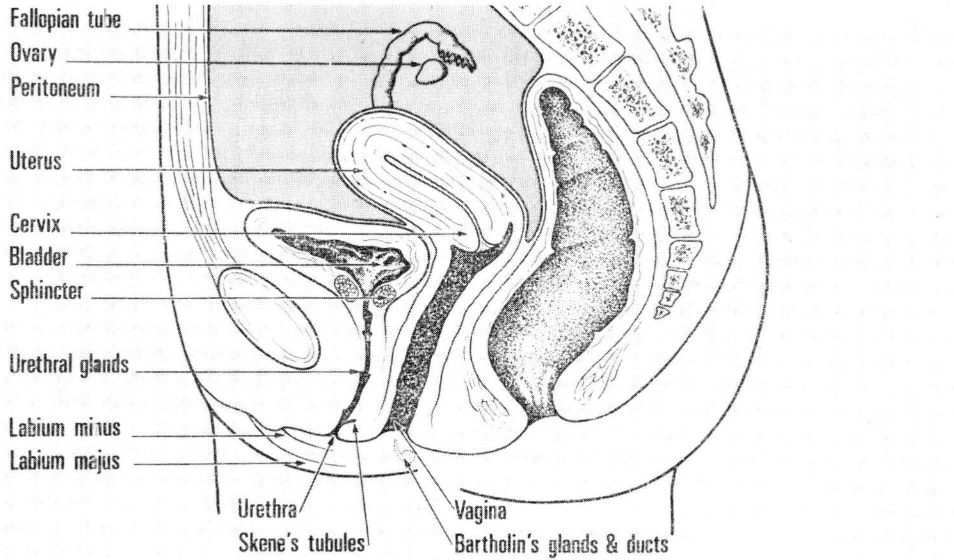

FIG. 113—Anatomical diagram of the female genito-urinary tract.

SYMPTOMS AND SIGNS

Gonorrhoea in men rarely is symptomless; commonly, some degree of *dysuria* occurs. A slight itching or burning on micturition is referred to the tip of the penis and the distal portion of the urethra. Occasionally dysuria is agonising and may be associated with nocturnal priapism or chordee. Increased *frequency* of micturition normally occurs first. Discharge begins in men with a slight mucoid or serous exudate which becomes heavily purulent or occasionally sanious. The lips of the urinary meatus become red, swollen and everted, and the urine in the first glass of the two-glass test becomes hazy from the presence of pus or shows the presence of purulent flakes. A slight, tender enlargement of the inguinal lymph glands may be noted.

Although women may complain of *dysuria* and *frequency*, more often symptoms are absent or they are slight and dismissed.

Urgency, haematuria or retention are rare in either sex. A low backache is not uncommon, together with some degree of ill-health. Vaginal discharge is noted, but is frequently said to be no worse than usual.

The primary sites of infection in men are the anterior third of the urethra, and in women the urethra and cervix. A careful examination is carried out and the specimens taken from the above sites to isolate the bacterium. In acute gonorrhoea in men, profuse purulent discharge from the urinary meatus is usually present. In the early stages the discharge is minimal; and in a number of patients the signs remain slight and 'stripping' of the urethra is necessary before taking specimens. In such cases it is useful to collect specimens in the morning before micturition. In a typical case the purulent discharge has a greeny yellow tinge. A loop-ful of discharge is spread on a glass slide; the smear is then stained by Gram's method (p. 202) and inspected under the microscope using a $\frac{1}{12}$th oil-immersion objective. In cases of doubt, cultures may also be made to confirm the presence of the gonococcus (p. 203). Sometimes a characteristic smell is present.

Apart from urethritis in men there may be signs of meatitis consisting of redness, oedema and ectropion, a secondary balanoposthitis, dorsal lymphangitis with oedema, and slight, tender bilateral lymph adenitis. The extent of urethral involvement in men is determined by the 'two-glass' urine test. The appearance of flakes and haze in the first glass alone indicates inflammation of the anterior two-thirds of the urethra. (See 'Urinary Inspection', p. 200).

In women the local appearances of acute infection vary greatly, from the normal for lower genito-urinary structures to signs of acute inflammation. Usually vulval signs are limited to slight discharge with injection of the urinary orifice. Uncommonly there is acute vulvitis (profuse discharge, reddening, excoriation and oedema of labia) together with oedema, reddening and discharge at the urinary meatus, and obvious involvement of Skene's tubules. As a rule the vagina contains some purulent exudate. The cervix in acute infection usually shows signs of inflammation, that is injection and congestion about the os, with or without an 'angry' erosion of the vaginal cervix. The secretion is mucopurulent. Sometimes purulent follicles are to be seen at an early stage on the crevix. Occasionally the first symptom is one of pelvic inflammation due to spread of the infection (p. 126).

The patient should lie, for preference, in the lithotomy position; after examination of the vulva and perineum, a smear and culture are taken first from the urethra. This is facilitated by 'stripping' the urethra from the inside of the vagina with the index finger, from behind forwards. A speculum is then passed and, after 'presenting' the cervix uteri, specimens of mucopus from within the cervical canal are obtained for both smear and culture.

Mucocutaneous manifestations are uncommon and consist of several well differentiated types of lesion. Local lesions, consisting of vesicles, pustules or small ulcerations, may occur on the skin or on moist epithelium of the genitalia. Probably some factor of irritation or surface maceration is necessary for this to occur. Rarely it complicates a suppurative lymphangitis. Erythemas of scarletiniform type or an erythema multiforme-like eruption may occur in acute or severe cases. In septicaemia the rash may be purpuric. A scarletiniform rash has been described in relation with gonorrhoeal rheumatism. Keratodermia (gonococcal hyperkeratosis) is seen likewise in this form of rheumatism; but it is now regarded as belonging more often than not to Reiter's syndrome, occurring in gonorrhoea where there may be a dual aetiology. It is only where untreated gonorrhoea is to be seen that absolute proof of this hypothesis of a dual aetiology is likely to be found (p. 154).

Spread of infection into the genito-urinary tract takes place at any time during the acute phase of the disease. In men this usually includes such structures as Littre's glands, lacunae of Morgagni, the subepithelial tissues, and later may include Cowper's glands, the prostate gland, the seminal vesicles, and the base of the bladder. When such spread occurs the urine contains larger flakes and threads (which indicate duct involvement) and the second glass of urine contains a greater degree of haze (p. 200).

Involvement of Skene's para-urethral glands occurs in women, with spread to the base of the bladder. Bartholin's glands may become involved, and the infection may ascend from the cervix into the endometrium and into the Fallopian tubes.

DIAGNOSIS

Stained films are prepared from the smears taken from urethra and cervix, using Gram's method. *The Neisseria gonorrhoeae* or 'gonococcus' is readily identified in the specimen from the male urethra as a 'Gram-negative diplococcus' (pink-stained and about 1 μ in diameter) lying in paired clusters within the leucocyte (indicating phagocytosis). Extracellular diplococci may be gonococcal but should not be accepted as such, especially in the presence of a mixed bacterial flora.

Smears from women usually contain leucocytes and epithelial cells with a confusing, mixed bacterial flora. Typical clusters of intracellular diplococci may be demonstrable, but this is far from being the rule. A good culture-technique is therefore very important when examining women for this infection, since it is also necessary to grow the organism if 'proof' of its nature is required, for example for any medico-legal purpose or in child infection. There are several different types in the group *Neisseria*, one of which is the gonococcus. The gonococcus is demonstrated by the 'fermentation' reaction of the organism after culture: it ferments glucose but not maltose. Immuno-fluorescent techniques are now employed to demonstrate the organism but will not replace the need for routine culture (p. 203). The bacterium is a delicate one; thus a medium for culture-work containing heated whole blood (chocolate blood agar) is commonly used (p. 203). The inoculated medium must be placed at once in an incubator at 37° C. in an atmosphere of diminished oxygen and increased carbon dioxide. A simple air-excluding tin containing a lighted candle is satisfactory.

DIFFERENTIAL DIAGNOSIS

Other causes of urethral inflammation and genital discharge must be excluded. These are discussed on p. 136.

THE GONOCOCCAL COMPLEMENT FIXATION TEST (p. 204)

Whilst the gonococcal complement fixation test (which detects specific antibody) is of some value in the investigation of persisting gonorrhoea, it is not absolutely dependable. The reaction is usually negative for 10–14 days following infection, and may remain negative during the entire course of uncomplicated gonorrhoea in men or women. A positive reaction is obtained in infection of the posterior urethra in men, and in local or systemic complications of either sex.

After infection has been eradicated, the complement fixation test gradually becomes negative in the course of six to eight weeks. In some cases the test remains positive after the cure of infection. The value of the gonococcal complement fixation test may be summed up: a single negative reaction is of no significance in early infection; a positive reaction indicates the possibility of past gonococcal infection or of an active un-eradicated focus of infection; but unfortunately a persistently positive result may also be of little importance. Titres above 1 : 2 are significant.

TREATMENT OF ACUTE GONORRHOEA

Antibiotic treatment of acute gonorrhoea is in most cases rapidly effective. During treatment, and until it is pronounced to be

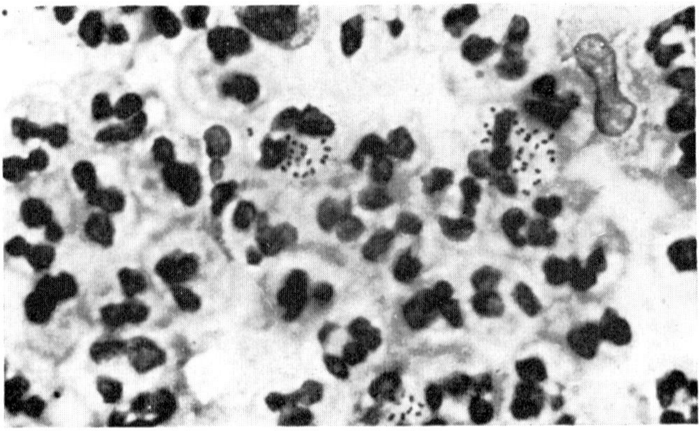

FIG. 114.

Neisseria gonorrhoeae from male urethra.

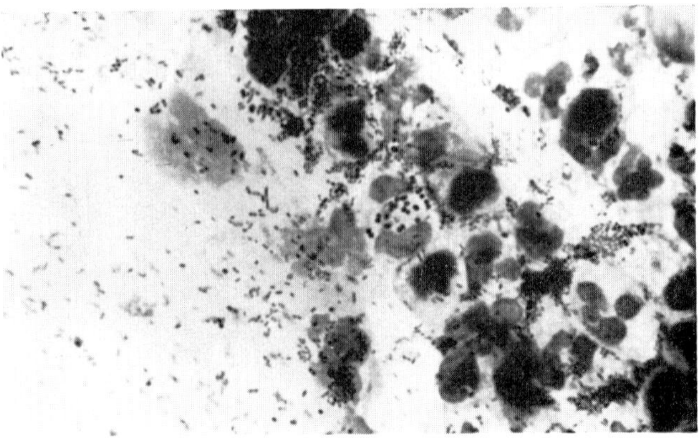

FIG. 115.

Neisseria gonorrhoeae from female cervix, illustrating the difficulty of picking out the intracellular diplococcus when a heavy nonspecific cocco-bacillary flora is also present.

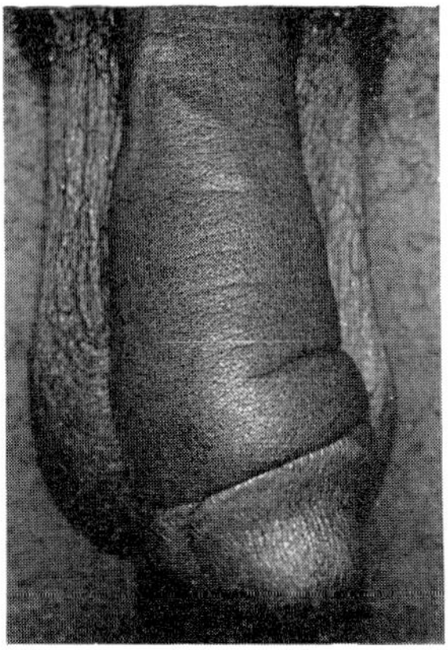

FIG. 116.

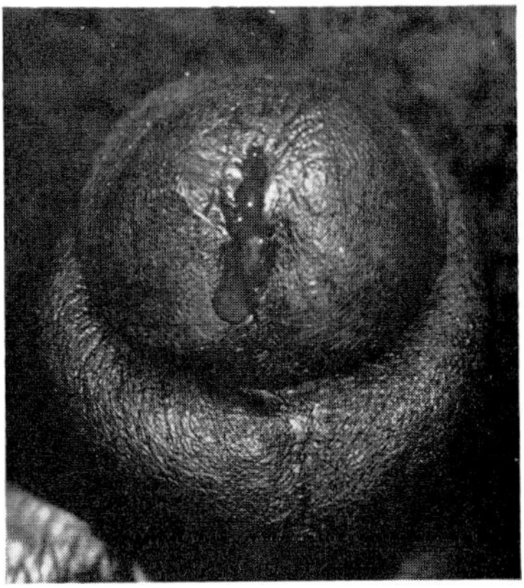

FIG. 117.

Purulent discharge with lymphoedema of prepuce and shaft of penis, in acute gonorrhoea.

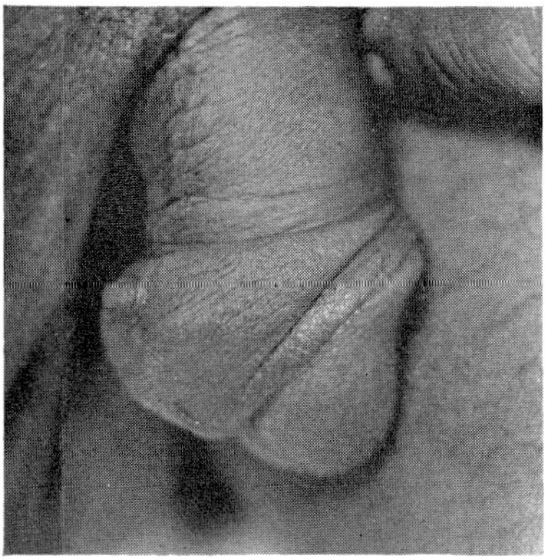

FIG. 118.

Tysonitis showing quite localised swelling.

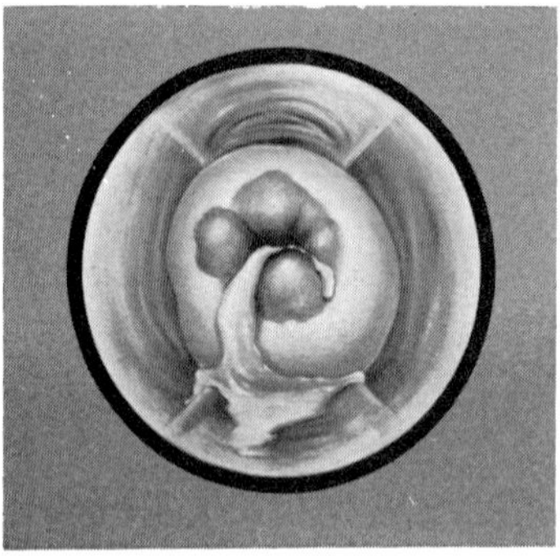

FIG. 119.

Cervicitis, showing purulent secretion, and inflammatory erosion.

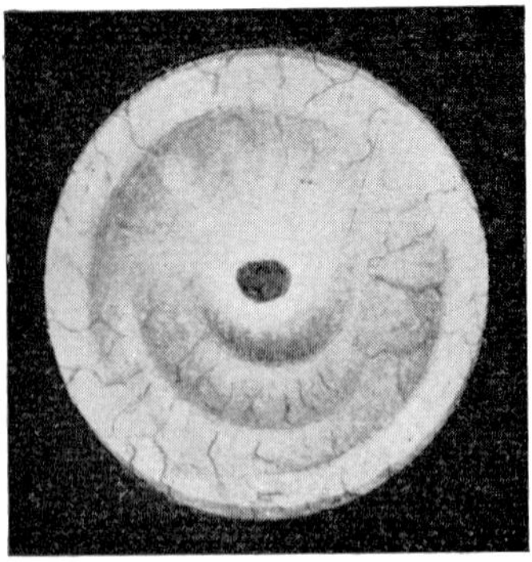

FIG. 120.

Stricture, showing the fibrotic ring unevenly contracted; the urethral epithelium is slightly inflamed.

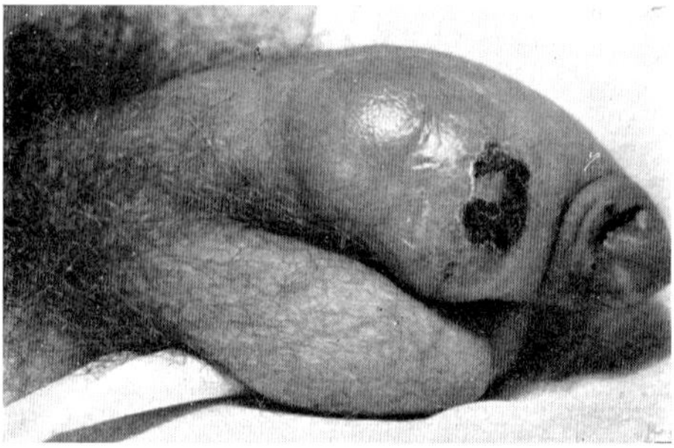

FIG. 121.

Peri-urethral abscess pointing subcutaneously in anterior penile urethra.

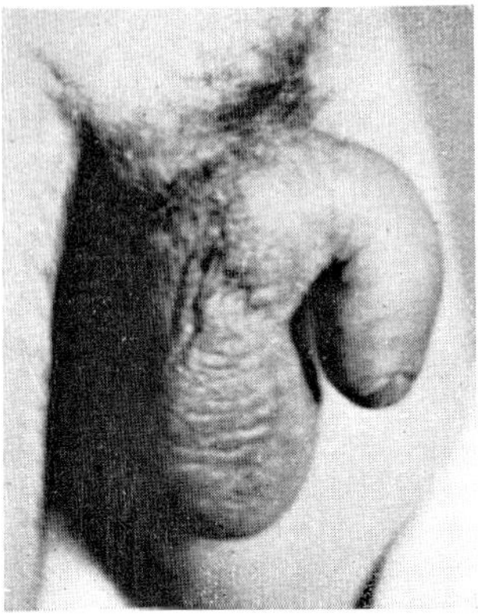

FIG. 122.

Peri-urethral abscess at peno-scrotal junction.

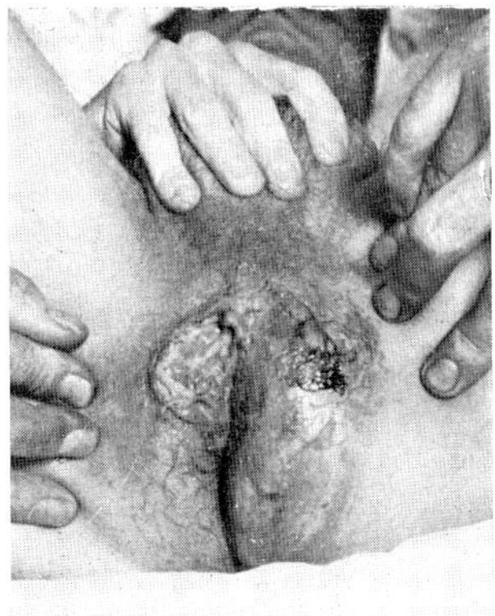

FIG. 123.

Spontaneous rupture of bilateral abscess of Cowper's Gland.

effective, the patient should consume over 3 litres of water daily, refrain from alcohol and sexual intercourse, and pay attention to such aspects of health as rest and sleep. Care should be taken over the disposal of toilet articles and discharges for the first 48 hours. Infection by non-sexual means is more likely to be transferred to young girls than to others.

The standard treatment for acute gonorrhoea is no less than three daily intramuscular injections of procaine penicillin G, of one million units each. This dose should be exceeded, and the course prolonged, when complications are present. If the organism is relatively resistant to penicillin, or if the patient is sensitised to the drug, another antibiotic, preferably tetracycline, is prescribed: 1 g. daily in divided dosage (0·25 g. q.d.s.) for four or five days. For optimal absorption to occur this drug must be taken outside meal-times. Erythromycin, 0·5 g. q.d.s. for four days, is useful, and kanamycin and trimethoprim may also be given.

An unsatisfactory response to penicillin is indicated by the persistence of urethral discharge or of flakes in the first glass of urine; but the gonococcus is usually not demonstrable in either, and does not reappear in the exudate for a further two or three days.

The rapid action of the successful antibiotic drugs in gonorrhoea makes local therapy, such as urethral irrigation, unnecessary. The patient is rendered non-infectious in 24–48 hours.

In an early case of uncomplicated infection (anterior urethritis) in men, the urinary meatus shows no sign of discharge from the third day after treatment, and the urine is clear in four to five days.

In women the infection is likely to be of longer standing, and in these circumstances a slightly prolonged course of therapy is desirable.

Persistent Infection

Failure of acute gonorrhoea to respond promptly to treatment may be due to one of several well defined causes: the organism itself may not be fully sensitive to the drug used; the patient may have failed to attend daily for the injections of antibiotic; or may have failed to take an oral antibiotic as prescribed; the patient may have indulged in alcohol or had further sexual contact with an infected person; the infection may have spread further into the tissues and adnexae of the genital tract, thus complicating the picture before treatment; presence of anatomical abnormalities such as meatal sinus or hypospadias; double infection (*e.g.* trichomonal, viral, mycoplasmal or mixed bacterial urethritis).

Criteria of Cure

These may be summarised as: absence of symptoms and signs; absence of gonococci in smears; negative cultures for gonococci in women; normal appearance of urine in men; negative gonococcal complement fixation test.

A period of observation of at least one month is necessary in men; and three negative cultures taken towards the end of each monthly period (when the cervical secretion is still more profuse) in women. Without a period of surveillance the criteria of cure of gonorrhoea are of less use. The organism may lie in the tissues, causing little or no detectable inflammatory response until relapse takes place. Response to treatment is more effectively assessed in men than in women, and it is in the latter that greater care is necessary before pronouncing a cure.

If there is a delayed or unsatisfactory response to treatment in the male, the prostate gland and its secretion should be examined (p. 142) and urethroscopy performed (p. 196).

A routine check for syphilis has to be made in all cases at an interval of three months. To exclude syphilis which may have been masked by penicillin used to treat gonorrhoea, a check at six months may have to be advised.

COMPLICATIONS OF GONORRHOEA

Complications arise from extension of the acute infection. Extension may occur locally into the tissues of the genito-urinary tract, or spread generally into other structures of the body via the blood stream. A second type of general complication results from a hyper-immune reaction and gives rise to rheumatism and arthritis in the patient.

LOCAL COMPLICATIONS IN MEN

Any of the local structures may be involved, *i.e.*: (1) *anteriorly*: subpreputial sac, paraurethral ducts, Tyson's glands; the lacunae of Morgagni, Littré's glands; the subepithelial tissue of any portion of the urethral tract; Cowper's ducts and glands. (2) *posteriorly*: prostatic ducts and glands, ejaculatory ducts and seminal vesicles, vasa deferentia and epididymes; the trigone of the bladder.

Complications *anteriorly* occur as part of a spread of infection and are not uncommon. A knowledge of the anatomy and a thorough examination of the parts directly and, if necessary, by urethroscopy, will reveal the anterior local lesions. Some lesions progress to abscess formation. Severe infection of the subepithelial tissues may result in peri-urethral abscess: this is especially liable to occur in the case of Littre's gland; infection results in blockage of its duct and abscess formation. The lesion should be suspected when there is an enlarging tender swelling in the spongiosum. Fibrous stricture formation occurs as a result of subepithelial infection. Contraction of the fibrous tissue of the stricture is slow, and it usually takes some 10–15 years for it to reach 'pin-hole' size.

Treatment of the anterior type of complication remains conservative: *i.e.* longer courses of antibiotics, procaine penicillin G intramuscularly, 1 mega-unit twice daily or daily for a week, local heat and local bathes or irrigation, gentle massage in order to drain the gland or focus, or massage over a urethral sound to obtain this effect. It is important to encourage drainage into the urethra rather than allow an inflamed gland to 'point' into the spongiosa and rupture externally.

Treatment of fibrous urethral stricture is by intermittent dilatation. Submucous infiltrations or 'soft' strictures may also require occasional dilatation. 'Whips' or gum-elastic bougies are used in small strictures, and subsequently curved metal sounds are introduced weekly or fortnightly until the lumen is thoroughly dilated. Chemotherapy or antibiotics should be used to keep the urine free from infection. A concomitant prostatitis must be treated.

Complications *posteriorly* are less common today when the patient is alert to infection, and therapy is usually effective in the acute phase. A number of years ago 70–80 per cent of cases of acute gonorrhoea presented with the posterior urethra already involved. Today this occurs in less than 10 per cent of cases. Posterior urethritis is sooner or later complicated by prostato-vesiculitis and not infrequently by epididymitis and cystitis. Constitutional symptoms such as malaise, headache, loss of appetite, and pyrexia make their appearance. Frequency, dysuria or haematuria occur. Pains radiate along the urethra to thighs, back, the suprapubic area, groins and, at times, upwards along the lines of the ureters, due to posterior urethritis and extension of inflammation into the prostate and seminal ducts.

Prostatitis

In acute or subacute prostatitis symptoms are similar to those described above. In addition the patient may have a sensation of heat, discomfort or swelling in the perineal region or rectum. The infection in the prostatic alveoli results in a tender, swollen lobe or lobes of the gland palpable by examination per rectum, commonly with defined areas of 'boggy' softening, which later become firm and nodular.

Should the inflammation proceed to abscess formation the symptoms and signs are more marked. There is a high pyrexia. Retention of urine may occur, and the gland felt 'per rectum' is large and soft. There is a danger of rupturing the abscess into the pelvic tissues by probing too firmly with the finger.

TREATMENT

The treatment of acute prostatitis consists in more prolonged antibiotic therapy (1 mega-unit procaine penicillin G intramuscularly twice daily until the temperature subsides and subsequently daily for a week to 10 days), and later gentle pressure upon, or massage of, the gland 'per rectum' to encourage drainage into the urethra, and general measures suited to the degree of illness. In acute cases there are constitutional symptoms and signs and the patient should rest in bed. Where there is an abscess direct palpation of the gland should be cautious. Hot hip-baths are useful. Retention of urine may yield to such measures but catheterization may be necessary.

The abscess usually ruptures spontaneously within 24–48 hours into the posterior urethra with immediate relief of symptoms Prostatic massage, which consists in drawing the index finger about five times across each lobe of the gland in turn, may now be instituted to speed up drainage. Surgical intervention is not required, but should be considered if there is a danger of rupture into the rectum or pelvic tissues.

In cases of subacute inflammation, a course of short-wave diathermy to the gland together with tetracycline 0·25 g. six-hourly for a week may assist resolution.

Cowperitis

This occasionally occurs as a sequel to posterior urethritis. Additional symptoms are pains extending into the rectum and thighs. The gland is only palpable either side of the median raphe of the perineum when inflamed. Treatment is with rest, antibiotics and local heat or hip-bathes.

Seminal Vesiculitis

This condition exists to an undetermined extent together with prostatitis and posterior urethritis. The symptoms of vesiculitis are vague: frequently a lower abdominal pain may be exacerbated by colonic movement or a full bladder, and somewhat relieved by defaecation and micturition. The vesicles are difficult to palpate in their normal healthy state; but when inflamed may be felt as small, tender, sausage-like structures above the prostate, which move away when palpated 'per rectum'. Treatment is by antibiotics and general measures.

Epididymitis

Involvement of the vas deferens and the epididymis arises from direct extension of gonococcal infection from a posterior urethritis with associated prostate-vesiculitis. Localisation of the infection in the epididymis is predisposed to by trauma, effort, by too vigorous prostato-vesicular massage, or by incorrect technique of posterior urethroscopy. Inflammatory swelling of the vas and epididymis seldom occurs before the second or third week of infection.

Symptoms frequently arise suggesting the impending involvement of the intra-scrotal structures. Pain in the groin, localised about the line of the lower third of the ureter, vaguely radiating along the line of the spermatic cord, or a feeling of weight in the testicle of the affected side, precedes the inflammatory swelling by 24–48 hours. These symptoms are followed by a painful sensation in the lower pole of the epididymis. On examination a small, hard, acutely tender nodule is detected before the inflammatory changes rapidly involve the entire epididymis, giving rise to a large tender inflammatory mass, which may almost completely encircle the body of the testis. The overlying scrotal skin becomes reddened, hot and tender, and there is a secondary hydrocoele with subcutaneous oedema. The symptoms become progressively severe and the temperature may reach 39·4°–40° C. (103°–104° F.). Urethral discharge becomes scanty or is absent. The condition is usually unilateral, the left side being the more frequently affected. The vas deferens may be simultaneously involved and show a hard, rigid, tender inflammatory swelling.

DIAGNOSIS

The occurrence of an acute inflammatory swelling of the epididymis or vas deferens in association with a gonococcal prostato-vesiculitis suggests the diagnosis. Other causes of the epididymitis may arise from non-gonococcal genito-urinary infections, for example *E. coli* (p. 136); metastatic infection in association with bacteraemia; tuberculosis. Consideration of these possibilities indicates the local, general and pathological investigation required in the individual patient.

Lesions of the epididymis may also have to be differentiated from swellings of the testis, like the orchitis in mumps, in which the associated urethral discharge may at first suggest gonorrhoea or neoplasm. They must also be distinguished from lesions of the scrotal contents such as hydrocoele, spermatocoele, varicocoele, and an inguinal hernia.

TREATMENT

This consists of rest in bed until pain has been relieved and the swelling is diminished. Local treatment, apart from a suspensory bandage, is seldom required. Antibiotic therapy is rapidly effective. Not infrequently a painful fibrous nodule may be left, usually to the lower pole of the epididymis, which takes from one to several months to disappear, or may remain for years.

Cystitis and Upper Urinary Tract Infection

In the male, gonococcal cystitis is now uncommon. The squamous epithelium of the bladder is resistant to this infection and involvement only occurs in the presence of a mixed bacterial infection, for example, of the gonococcus and *E. coli*. The changes are commonly limited to the trigone of the bladder and are seldom generalised.

Additional symptoms when the bladder is involved are suprapubic tenderness and a feeling of weight in the pelvis. In the three-glass urine test all the specimens are turbid, at times the urine being uniformly bloodstained. This contrasts with the terminal bleeding of acute posterior urethritis. The diagnosis is in the majority of cases inferential, since catheterisation is undesirable.

Pyelitis and pyelonephritis may arise from direct extension of infection from gonococcal cystitis, or may be metastatic. The gonococcus is rarely solely responsible for the infection; secondary organisms, staphylococci, streptococci and *E. coli* are commonly present. Such complications are unlikely to occur nowadays.

The treatment does not differ from that for all bacterial infections of the renal tract: rest, alkaline fluid intake and suitable antibiotics.

LOCAL COMPLICATIONS IN WOMEN

It is important to realise that local complications are more common in women than in men, due largely to the fact that women harbour the bacterium of the disease for longer periods without treatment.

Urethral

Skene's tubules may be persistent foci of infection, but this is much less common today. Antibiotics, and massage over a sound to promote drainage, is all that is required as treatment. Skenitis almost never results in stricture.

Bartholinitis

The occurrence of an acute inflammatory swelling (red, warm, tender) in the posterior half of the labium majus points to an involvement of the gland. It is usually unilateral. Abscess formation results in more pronounced pain and signs of inflammatory swelling.

Chronic bartholinitis may yield to conservative treatment. In many cases however surgical removal of the gland becomes necessary in order to avoid recurrent inflammation. Probing the duct in order to restore patency is not often successful.

A Bartholin cyst results from blockage of the lumen of the duct, resulting from previous inflammation. Its presence may cause pain and local tenderness, which becomes more exquisite at the onset of infection. It has to be distinguished from the lymphatic oedema of the labium accompanying a primary syphilitic sore. The cyst may have to be removed when there is recurrent infection.

Endometritis and Metritis

Endometritis is rarely met with in practice; this is probably due to its being masked by the symptoms and signs of the accompanying endocervicitis and salpingitis.

Acute endometritis is accompanied by menstrual dysfunction and a profuse, thin, purulent or sanious cervical discharge (thinner than in cervicitis alone). The uterus is enlarged and tender. There is sacral and supra-pubic pain and constitutional symptoms are present sometimes with a marked rise of temperature nausea and vomiting.

Salpingitis

Infection of the Fallopian tubes takes place by direct extension of the disease from the endocervix. Premonitory symptoms and signs may occur, such as pain at the menstrual period, menorrhagia, the passage of clots, and lower abdominal pain or discomfort. The onset of acute salpingitis is accompanied by severe pain in the lower abdomen, sharp rise of temperature to 39°–39·4° C. (102°–103° F.), malaise, nausea and vomiting. There is *bilateral* tenderness with muscle spasm, low in the abdomen, which is more marked on one side. In acute cases the pain is often colicky in nature and may be felt in the vulva. On bi-manual examination the uterus feels tender and may be enlarged. There is also acute tenderness in the lateral fornices. A definite tubal swelling can be made out after the first few days, usually on one or the other side.

Pelvic peritonitis is common in this condition, the symptoms being overshadowed by the salpingitis. Generalised peritonitis rarely occurs in adults.

Subacute salpingitis is very prone to develop in untreated gonorrhoea in women. The symptoms are pain and discomfort in the lower abdomen, dyspareunia and mild malaise. There is, more often than not, slight abnormality of the periods with increase of symptoms. The rise of temperature is intermittent. Bi-manual palpation reveals tenderness in the lateral fornices, with the presence of tubal thickening, or a definite mass predominantly on one side.

DIAGNOSIS

Evidence of lower abdominal symptoms and signs associated with pyrexia and gonococcal cervicitis suggest the diagnosis of salpingitis. In the absence of a diagnosis of gonorrhoea, other causes of inflammation have to be considered such as ovarian endometriosis, ectopic pregnancy, appendicitis, tuberculous salpingitis or pyelitis. Endometriosis is suggested by the timing of the pains, which occur during and just after the period, and may be accompanied by brief pyrexia. Ectopic pregnancy is suggested by the lack of the expected period, followed some days later by persistent slight bleeding per vaginam, collapse and abdominal distension which may be accompanied by pyrexia. The pain of appendicitis is usually more central, and there are bowel symptoms or nausea present; that of pyelitis is more lateral and radiating from the renal angle into the groin, together with pronounced dysuria and frequency. A dilation and curettage may have to be performed to exclude tuberculous infection.

TREATMENT AND PROGNOSIS

Rest in bed and antibiotic treatment speedily bring down the temperature and reduce the acute inflammation. The organism disappears from the cervix. Penicillin, one million units of the procaine salt (together with benzylpenicillin if deemed necessary in a severe case) is injected intramuscularly, at first twice daily until the temperature falls and subsequently daily, for a week or 10 days. In the subacute to chronic type of illness or when recovery appears to be incomplete, short-wave diathermy radiation to the pelvic viscera together with penicillin, or with tetracycline 0·5 g. six-hourly is beneficial.

Persistent pain, discomfort or dyspareunia is not uncommon after treatment of this condition, especially in severe cases and those which have not been treated early. Infertility due to permanent blockage of the tubes may occur. Tubal insuflation should then be undertaken. Greater attention to general health factors and a convalescent holiday are helpful in difficult cases in promoting a final cure.

Upper Urinary Tract Infection—*see* p. 124.

VULVO-VAGINITIS IN CHILDREN

The term vulvo-vaginitis includes a number of prepubertal infections which vary greatly in their aetiology, symptoms and clinical signs. Epidemics may occur amongst children in institutions. Neisserian infection in such cases is not always due to *N. gonorrhoeae*.

Direct infection may occur from criminal assault, precocious sexual intercourse, or perversions; rarely *in utero* or during the process of birth. Indirect means of conveying infection are infected bedclothes, towels, nurses' aprons, chamber pots, and rectal thermometers, all of which have been incriminated.

Vulvo-vaginitis may be classified as: bacterial, trichomonal, viral, and mycotic. The relative incidence today is, very approximately: (1) Bacteria: neisserian—gonococcal and non-gonococcal, 3 per cent; others—staphylococci (pathogenic and nonpathogenic), streptococci, enterococci, *E. coli* and coliforms, proteus, 75 per cent. (2) Trichomonas vaginalis, 2 per cent. (3) Candida, 4 per cent. (4) Others, 16 per cent.

Certain factors predispose to infection: for example, chronic local uncleanliness, dirty clothing, chronic masturbation, foreign bodies in the vagina or thread-worm infestation of the bowel.

In vulvo-vaginitis before puberty, infection is almost invariably limited to the vulva, vagina and urethra. At birth there is at first an adult type of vaginal mucosa due to oestrogens absorbed from the maternal circulation. Within three months the oestrogens disappear from the infant's circulation and the mucosa becomes thin and composed of cubical cells, devoid of glycogen. The secretion is by now scanty and alkaline. It remains in this state until puberty, when the adult development of the genitalia and mucous membrane occurs. The non-involvement of the cervix and of the Bartholin glands in prepubertal infection must be attributed to the functional under-development of these organs.

The symptoms and signs vary from trivial to severe. Dysuria, increased frequency of micturition, and local irritation are present in varying degree. There may be retention of urine, and acute or subacute lower abdominal pain which may be confused with appendicitis. On examination, vulval inflammation or redness is observed with some degree of oedema, which may extend along the inner aspect of the thighs. Vaginal discharge is present. The urethra is involved in most instances. In the chronic cases clinical findings are often minimal or intermittent, and there is the danger that such cases may be the cause of an epidemic in an institution or ward for children.

COMPLICATIONS

Proctitis may result from direct spread of infection. Cervicitis occurs in a few cases. Extension of the gonococcal infection to the endometrium, Fallopian tubes, or pelvic peritoneum rarely occurs but remains a special danger with gonococcal infection.

TREATMENT

The condition in the child is treated in the same manner as in the adult, using a specific drug in suitable dosage for age and weight, together with a suitable period of observation, depending on the aetiology of infection.

For gonorrhoea, treatment consists of three or four daily intramuscular injections of procaine penicillin of at least 50,000 units per kg. weight daily dosage; or phenethicillin 0·25 g. six-hourly by mouth for four days. If the organism is less sensitive to penicillin, tetracycline is given in a daily dosage of 20 mg. kg.

weight. Its effect on dental enamel and bone must be remembered (p. 210).

GONOCOCCAL PROCTITIS

Gonococcal contamination of the anal canal and of the rectum is not infrequent in adult women with genital gonorrhoea, and in association with the vulvo-vaginitis in pre-pubertal girls. Infection can take place and is due to spread of infection from genital gonorrhoea. There is no definite evidence, however, that reinfection of the genital tract in women occurs from this source. In men the condition may rarely follow the rupture of a prostatic abscess, and abscess of Cowper's gland, or a posterior peri-urethral abscess. It occurs commonly as a direct infection in the homosexual.

SYMPTOMS AND SIGNS

The condition can be asymptomatic and may be detected only on careful routine examination. In many cases, however, patients complain of itching and a feeling of irritation around the anal orifice or formication over the inner aspect of the buttocks and perineum. In men, an acute proctitis causes pain in the rectum, abdominal discomfort, discharge and rectal tenesmus. Examination may reveal no apparent external signs; usually, however, there is some degree of peri-anal inflammation and a mucopurulent discharge either exudes or can be expressed from the anus. In cases of acute inflammation proctoscopy reveals a livid red mucous membrane coated with mucopus.

DIAGNOSIS

The occurrence during the course of a gonococcal infection of even vague symptoms referable to the rectum should lead to a careful local inspection, and to the bacteriological examination of any discharge. The ultimate confirmation of a diagnosis of gonococcal proctitis depends on the demonstration of the gonococcus in smear and, if necessary, in culture. Other conditions such as non-specific proctitis, lymphogranuloma venereum in women, regional enteritis or ulcerative colitis involving the rectum, should be excluded.

TREATMENT

To effect a cure proctitis requires longer treatment than does an acute genital infection. Following treatment the majority of cases rapidly clear up. Rarely, however, in the untreated case, ulceration of the mucous membrane, fissure-in-ano or perianal abscess may occur. If the condition has persisted untreated for a long time, submucous infiltration may lead to rectal stricture. Treatment is then on general surgical principles, after the appropriate measures have been taken to control the gonococcal infection. Non-specific proctitis may be treated by the insertion of e.g., organic arsenical rectal suppositories.

GONOCOCCAL OPHTHALMIA

The eye may be involved at any time during the course of a gonococcal infection by transfer of infective material from the genito-urinary focus, or as a systemic complication. In the newborn child, infection of the conjunctival sac, *ophthalmia neonatorum*, results from direct inoculation during the act of birth. Gonococcal inflammations may be of two kinds: (1) gonococcal ophthalmia, due to implantation of the bacterium, or (2) toxic inflammation caused by an hyperallergic phenomenon in the eye; in this type the organism is *not* present in the eye.

Ophthalmia Neonatorum

This is defined as 'any inflammation of the eyes in an infant accompanied by a purulent discharge from the eyes, occurring within twenty-one days from the date of birth'. It is notifiable in the United Kingdom.

Ophthalmia neonatorum may be due to the gonococcus or to other organisms. In the past the gonococcus was responsible for approximately two-thirds of all cases. In recent years, however, the condition has become uncommon. Associated with this disorder are the virus *C. oculogenitale*, the *Staphylococcus pyogenes* and a number of other bacteria.

In a gonococcal infection, inflammatory signs are present by the third or fourth day. In cases due to other organisms the incubation period generally varies from seven to twenty days. The longer the incubation period, the more likelihood there is of a mild infection with little risk of corneal damage.

The earliest sign to appear is a transverse reddening of the conjunctiva of the upper eyelid. This is rapidly followed by generalised injection, tumefaction and a sero-purulent discharge. As the condition progresses the eyelids become red and swollen, and there is a purulent, often sanious discharge from the conjunctival sac. Oedema of the upper lid may be so extensive as to cause it to overlap the lower lid. In the absence of treatment the cornea assumes a ground-glass appearance, and ulceration occurs. In fulminating cases the cornea would perforate in twenty-four to thirty-six hours with escape of the aqueous and prolapse of the iris. Impairment or complete loss of sight may result from leucoma, panophthalmitis, or secondary glaucoma. The condition is commonly mild and these complications are now rare.

TREATMENT OF GONOCOCCAL OPHTHALMIA

Parenteral penicillin is rapidly curative. Local therapy is restricted to normal saline bathes or the use of very mild antiseptics. The only antibiotic which should be used locally is $\frac{1}{2}$ per cent chloramphenicol.

The best prevention is the discovery and cure of infection in the expectant mother.

GENERAL COMPLICATIONS IN MEN AND WOMEN

Metastatic Complications

Gonorrhoea usually remains a localised genito-urinary disease. In certain cases, now uncommon in this country, with acute or chronic involvement of the prostate and vesicles in the male, or of the cervix and uterine tubes in the female, the gonococcus may enter the blood stream and cause metastatic infection of other structures. Such metastatic lesions are usually restricted to those involving the joints and tendon sheaths. These manifestations occur about the third or fourth week of untreated infection, but may appear as early as the first week or be delayed until the seventh or even the tenth week. Septicaemia is now unknown.

The joint manifestations may be acute, diffuse arthritis (monoarticular), acute polyarthritis or subacute or chronic, hydrops articuli.

Diffuse Arthralgia and Acute Arthritis

Pain is the prominent feature of diffuse gonococcal arthralgia, and tends to move from joint to joint. No other clinical features may be apparent except slight reddening and increased temperature of the skin over the affected joint(s). The history of shifting joint pains suggests acute polyarticular rheumatism. Gonococcal arthralgia, however, fails to respond to the administration of salicylates, and the temperature is seldom so high as in acute rheumatic fever. The symptoms and signs of genital gonococcal infection should point to the suspected diagnosis.

Acute arthritis is often limited to a single large joint, and commonly occurs during or after a stage of diffuse arthralgia. The joints involved, in order of frequency, are the knee, ankle, wrist, shoulder, hip and elbow. The joint rapidly becomes swollen, extremely tender to touch, active or passive movements being resisted because of pain. The overlying skin is red and tense, and there is a marked increase of local temperature. The swelling is due to a sero-fibrinous then purulent exudate into the joint cavity, the synovial membrane, and the peri-synovial structures. The tendons, ligaments and bursae in relation to the affected joint may also be involved. Acute arthritis is accompanied by constitutional symptoms, the temperature frequently varying between 38° and 39·4° C. (100° and 103° F.). In such cases the bacterium is present in the joint exudate. The gonococcal complement fixation test is usually positive.

Gonorrhoeal Rheumatism

Certain systemic complications of gonorrhoea can occur without the organism being present in the particular exudates or secretions of the structures involved.

The organism has never been isolated, for example, from the lesion of iritis accompanying an attack of gonorrhoea, unless the organism has also been implanted in the eye by a finger, etc. These manifestations of conjunctivitis or iritis have long been known to be commonly associated with a vague flitting arthritis, polyarthritis or tenosynovitis. Iritis is seen almost exclusively in men (p. 131). Since the eye lesions exacerbate with fresh attacks of gonorrhoea (or the use of gonococcal vaccines in days gone-by), it is considered that a 'rheumatism' can be directly related to gonorrhoea as an allergic phenomenon.

Most of the patients today, in the United Kingdom, showing evidence of a polyarthritic syndrome occurring during an attack of gonorrhoea are considered to be cases of a Reiter's syndrome. Nevertheless, this is not the experience of observers in all parts of the world, especially where gonorrhoea is seen as an untreated disease. The manifestations of gonorrhoeal rheumatism when they occur are similar to those of Reiter's syndrome, which is described on p. 154.

Treatment

Metastatic and allergic gonococcal complications require: (1) treatment of the genital infection, and (2) general or particular measures directed towards the patient's general illness and the local lesions. The treatment of arthritis and of ocular lesions is discussed under Reiter's syndrome (p. 164). The local genital infection is treated on the same lines as the local complications of acute gonorrhoea.

Penicillin should be given to all patients with general complications, by intramuscular injection, 1 million units of procaine penicillin G twice daily for a few days while the temperature is raised, and subsequently daily for a week.

SELECTED BIBLIOGRAPHY

Bacteriology and Experimental Work

COLONIAL MORPHOLOGY AND VARIATION

Kellogg, D. S., Cohen, I. R., Norins, L. C., Schroeter, A. L. & Reising, G. (1968). *J. Bact.* **96,** 596.

L-FORM N. GONORRHOEAE

Roberts, D. B. (1966). *J. Bact.* **92,** 1609.

CULTURE MEDIUM

Thayer, J. D. & Martin, J. E. (1966). *Publ. Hlth Rep. Wash.* **81,** 559.

Wilkinson, A. E. (1965). *Br. J. vener. Dis.* **41,** 60.

SERUM ANTIBODY RESPONSE IN EXPERIMENTAL DISEASE

Cohen, I. R., Kellogg, D. S. & Norins, L. C. (1968). In press.

Identification by Immunofluorescent Method

Lind, I. (1967). *Acta path. microbiol. scand.* **70,** 613.

Sommerville, R. G. (1968). *WHO Vener. dis. trans.* (*gon.*) No. 23.

Control

Willcox, R. R. (1967). *Acta derm.-vener., Stockh.* **47,** 65.

Antibiotic Sensitivity of N. gonorrhoeae

WHO SCREENING CENTRE

Reyn, A. & Bentzou, M. W. (1968). *Br. J. vener. Dis.* **44,** 140.

CHAPTER 8

Non-Gonococcal Inflammatory Discharges and Non-Specific Urethritis

URETHRITIS IN MEN

Following sexual intercourse, inflammatory reactions of the urethra in men may result from several causes, infective and non-infective; none the less the aetiology in many instances remains unknown.

An inflammatory reaction in the male urethra, whether due to a so-called non-specific urethritis or to urethritis having a definite aetiology, carries with it a certain risk of local and general complications, and requires care in examination and treatment. The causes may be classified as:—

(1) *Specific infective*:

Virus:	*C. oculogenitale*	
Mycoplasma:	'T' strain	varying parasitism
	M. hominis strains	
Bacterium:	*N. gonorrhoeae*	
	Strept. faecalis	
	E. coli, and others.	
Yeast-like:	*Candida albicans*, and others.	
Protozoon:	*Trichomonas vaginalis*	

(2) *Non-Specific Urethritis*

The term excludes known infective causes and inflammations listed above and below under (1) and (3). This large group, known as non-specific urethritis, appears to be due to an acute or subacute inflammatory response brought about either by an 'ultramicroscopic' infecting agent not yet isolated, or by idiosyncratic factors connected with the tissues or their secretions, which result in an altered tissue reactivity, (*e.g.* allergy to vaginal or cervical secretions or products).

(3) *Other Causes of Urethral Inflammation*

Syphilis (either intrameatal chancre or intrameatal lesions of early stage of rash); chancroid; intrameatal genito-urinary tuberculosis; sequel to severe cystitis; foreign bodies inserted, or sequel to intrumentation; irritation from chemicals, antiseptics or contraceptives; sensitisation (allergy) to chemicals; urethral discharge as part of a general virus disease such as measles, mumps or hepatitis; urethritis due (rarely) to the less common bacteria (*e.g.* diphtheria), spirochaetes, protozoa or metazoa; urethritis secondary to virus papilloma or neoplastic lesion. Urethritis can also appear as the presenting symptom of a lower genito-urinary focus of infection, for example prostatitis, or urethral stricture.

Non-specific Urethritis

Since the condition of *non-specific urethritis* may have several causes, it is not surprising to find a variable clinical picture. In the acute type the discharge may be thick, with all the features of an acute abacterial urethritis. Usually, however, the condition is subacute, and either mucoid, muco-purulent or serous. Occasionally it is blood-stained or accompanied by haematuria: many, but not all, of these latter cases are due to *E. coli* infection; some are possibly due to mycoplasma; a few have a 'cobblestone' appearance in the epithelium; others may be due to a virus infection.

The symptoms can begin soon after coitus in the acute type, but more often the incubation period is two weeks or longer. Some patients note only frequency of micturition, irritation or discomfort, the discharge being brought to light on examination. In these mild cases a meatal specimen contains a mixed saprophytic bacterial flora. The urethra is injected to a variable degree and extent. The typical 'cobblestone' appearance described by Welsch is of uncertain significance.

The *diagnosis* depends upon the presence of polymorpho-nuclear leucocytes in the smear and the exclusion of known specific organisms. The appearance of the pus in the stained smear, especially of subacute cases, usually differs from that of acute

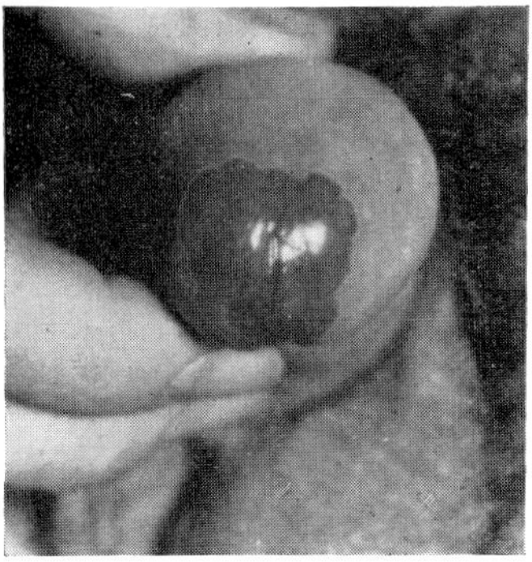

FIG. 124.

Acute circum-meatal balanitis in non-specific urethritis.

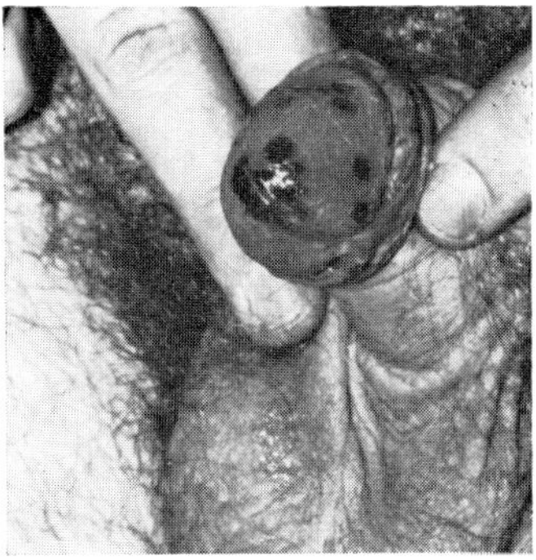

FIG. 125.

Circinate balanitis in non-specific urethritis.

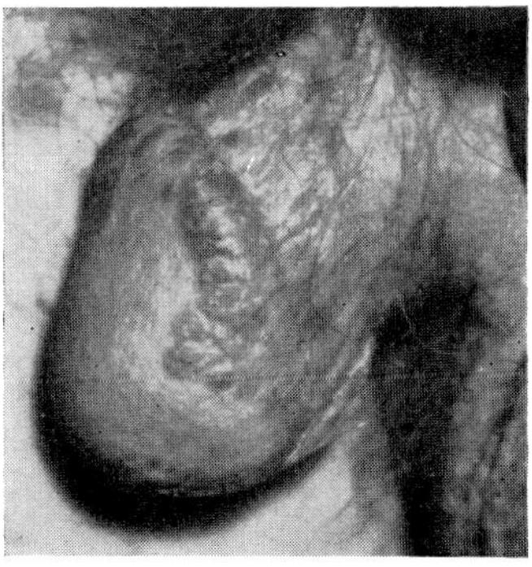

FIG. 126.

Chronic balanitis with features of keratodermia blenorrhagica.

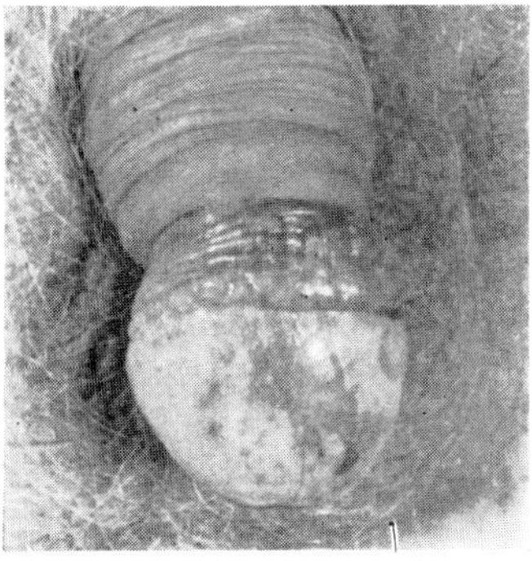

FIG. 127.

Thrush balanitis, showing typical maculopapular erosive lesions.

gonorrhoea in that the leucocytes are less clear in outline, less heavily stained, and are distributed amongst epithelial cells and mucus. A careful history and examination will exclude other and antecedent causes of dysuria and discharge, such as *stricture* of the urethra or *prostatitis*. Examination of the prostatic secretion is advisable in any patient of middle age, in one with a past history of urethritis, or in whom lower genito-urinary symptoms persist. A diagnosis of posterior urethritis or stricture should be confirmed by urethroscopy.

Specific Infective Urethritis other than Gonorrhoea

This may be due to a virus, *C. oculogenitale* (TRIC agent) (p. 1). Infection probably occurs in about 10 per cent of cases. Urethral smears, stained with Wright or Giemsa stain, will show epithelial inclusions in the majority of these cases; such inclusions are hard to find and must be distinguished from those due to mycoplasma. The virus may be grown on chick embryo. This viral urethritis, after a moderately short incubation period, presents as a meatitis with oedema, and later small, rounded yellowy-pink elevations of the epithelium which contain the inclusion bodies.

The role of the various strains of *mycoplasma* and whether they cause genito-urinary inflammation, still remains uncertain. Moderately high serum antibody titres however can accompany their presence, and they have occasionally been cultured from focal genital abscesses. Special, enriched media are required for their culture. The urethritis is of the acute or subacute variety. The organism is inhibited by tetracycline but not by erythromycin in clinical dosages; and it is apparent that a significant proportion of patients with a non-bacterial inflammation clinically respond to treatment with tetracycline when they do not do so to erythromycin or to penicillin.

Trichomonas Urethritis

The previous incidence of this infection was about 10 per cent in all cases of abacterial urethritis in men; this incidence is now decreasing. Appearances vary from a near-normal meatus and urethra to a condition of acute urethral inflammation with a

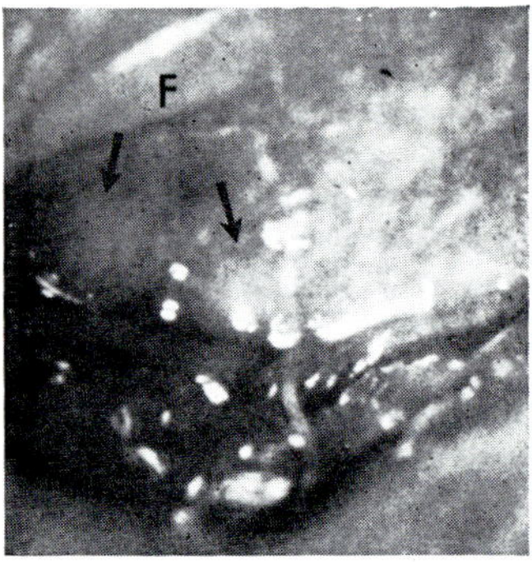

FIG. 128.
Inclusion meatitis.

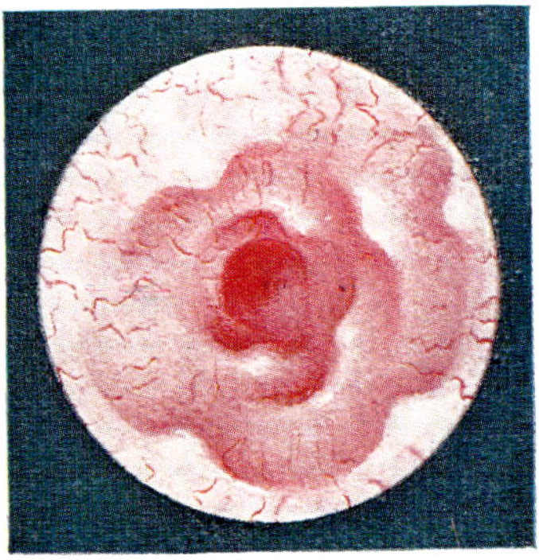

FIG. 129.
Follicular urethritis (Littré follicles).

frothy cream-coloured discharge. The latter appearance however is not very common. The presence of the protozoon is confirmed by gentle but firm scraping of the urethral wall with a loop, after instilling a few drops of normal saline into the lumen with a pipette, and examining the specimens by the hanging-drop (preferably dark-ground) method. Culture of the organism in a suitable medium, such as Feinberg or Wittington, increases the likelihood of diagnosis. The diagnosis is not easy in men, and it is advisable to examine the patient's female sexual partner in whom the presence of the trichomonas is easier to detect.

Thrush

This is common today in both the genital and alimentary tracts. A low-grade urethritis and balano-posthitis in men not infrequently accompanies a genital candidasis in their consorts. A urethral smear or smear prepared from centrifuged urinary deposit and stained with Gram stain contains either yeasts or hyphae, or both.

COURSE AND COMPLICATIONS

Non-specific urethritis tends to clear up spontaneously and rapidly in only a few instances; a large proportion (70–80 per cent) of cases respond well to tetracycline, less to streptomycin, and a few cases to sulphonamides. A number however are improved by therapy but continue to show inflammatory desquamations (purulent epithelial flakes) in the urine for about 4 to 6 weeks.

Local complications are similar to but milder than those occurring in gonorrhoea. Prostato-vesiculitis often occurs, especially with trichomonas urethritis. Fibrous stricture is rare, though soft infiltrations are not so infrequent. Epididymitis is less common. Involvement of the bladder and ureters occasionally occurs, resulting in abacterial cystitis or pyelonephritis. The clinical features of these conditions are as described in the section on gonococcal complications (p. 120).

TREATMENT

Non-Specific Urethritis

The usual treatment is tetracycline 1·0 g. daily in divided dosage for five days. The wide-spectrum antibiotic is used as a general antibacterial and antimycoplasmal measure. This régime, together with a liberal fluid intake helps a high proportion of patients. Further antibiotic treatment of those who do not respond is rarely successful, and the condition may not resolve in less than six weeks.

Specific Urethritis

This is treated with the drug appropriate to the condition. For *trichomonal* infections, Flagyl (metronidazole) 200 mg. is administered by mouth eight-hourly for seven days. For urethral or bladder *thrush* there is no proven specific oral therapy, and attempts to flush away the yeast through liberal fluid intake should be adopted. Nifuratel, however, by mouth, 200 mg. eight-hourly for a week, may be tried.

Amphotericin in solutin as a bladder-wash when the need arises can be helpful.

Viral Infection

Tetracycline 0·25 g. *q.d.s.* for 10 days is the treatment of choice. *Mycoplasma* responds readily to a smaller total dose of tetracycline.

Bacterial Urethritis

A wide-spectrum antibiotic such as tetracycline 0·25 g. *q.d.s.* for five days or any other suitable antibiotic is advocated (see Ch. 13); or trimethoprim 80 mg. *plus* sulphamethoxazole 0·5 g. *q.d.s.* for five days can be used (septrin.).

PROSTATITIS

Acute, or subacute, prostatitis and vesiculitis were common in a persisting gonococcal infection before the introduction of specific treatment. Subacute infection is now commoner as a sequel to non-specific urethritis and trichomonas urethritis. The condition is usually insidious in onset, attention being drawn to it by the persistence or recurrence of signs and symptoms of lower genito-urinary tract inflammation. The urine is often clear but it may contain large or small threads, the latter denoting a glandular duct inflammation. The symptoms may be diverse (p. 121) being the result of inflammation of the posterior urethra, ducts, and of the gland itself. Some degree of seminal vesiculitis usually accompanies the prostatitis.

DIAGNOSIS

This is made by expression of the prostatic secretion (after 'massage' of the prostate per rectum) and examining it. The nodularity, consistency and tenderness of the gland, as found by palpation are important signs. The secretion normally contains amorphous material (using an acid stain only such as carbol fuchsin) with deeper staining spherical bodies, the 'corpora amylacea'. There are normally few other cells present, and only the occasional leucocyte. A profusion of leucocytes in the prostatic secretion obtained *after* the patient has micturated, or 'clumps' of leucocytes, indicate inflammation. Occasionally the *Trichomonas vaginalis* will be found in the prostatic secretion. Its presence may be commoner than experience admits. Bacterial culture is often either negative or yields commensals. There is to date no evidence that a mycoplasma has a rôle, and studies with respect to the TRIC virus are not conclusive.

TREATMENT AND PROGNOSIS

Treatment consists in emptying the gland by massage of each lobe per rectum (p. 195). A recommended régime is massage two or three times weekly for four weeks, accompanied by short-wave diathermy directed to the gland, and antibiotics. A wide-spectrum antibiotic, such as tetracycline 0·25 g. six-hourly is initially given for seven days; followed by 1 g. by mouth, or intramuscular injections of tetracycline (0·2 g.) or of streptomycin (1 g.), at the time of massage. The disappearance of the leucocytes from the secretion and improvement in symptoms and signs follow in most cases.

In addition the effect of trypsin enzyme by mouth, 200,000 units daily in divided dosage, for a week at a time, may be tried together with the antibiotic. There is a greater chance of permanent improvement in the younger patient. In others the condition tends to relapse after a variable interval.

Although certain forms of rheumatism, especially uveitis and arthritis in men (for example, Reiter's syndrome and some cases of spondylitis), appear to be related to the presence of a lower genito-urinary infection and in particular of subacute prostatitis (p. 154), the majority of cases of prostatitis once diagnosed and treated do not seem to develop such a complication.

BALANOPOSTHITIS

Inflammation of the non-keratinised epithelium covering the glans penis is known as balanitis; that affecting the inner aspect of the prepuce is known as posthitis. Usually both structures are involved. Various bacteria, fusiform bacilli, Vincent's organisms and several spirochaetes tend to flourish in unhealthy conditions of the subpreputial sac.

AETIOLOGY

The causes of the condition may be summarised as follows:

1. *Local non-infective*: resulting from trauma, indiscriminate use of antiseptics (*e.g.* 'Dettol'), chemical soaps (*e.g.* tar),

sensitivity to various substances (*e.g.* contraceptive chemicals or sheaths) and various dermatoses (p. 168).

2. *Local infective*: (*a*) any of the causes of urethritis (p. 136) may result in a balanitis at the same time or it may occur with the ocular and arthritic manifestations of Reiter's syndrome; (*b*) discrete lesions due to organisms which result in sores (Part 1), and others, (Part 3), the commoner being herpes simplex, thrush and scabies.

3. *Constitutional*: (*a*) smegma, if left for long periods, may result in irritation, erosion and secondary infection; (*b*) glycosuria; (*c*) dermatoses (p. 168); (*d*) mucocutaneous syndromes, erythema multiforme (p. 176); Behçet's syndrome (p. 147); Stevens-Johnson syndrome (p. 176); Reiter's syndrome (p. 154).

4. *Neoplastic*: especially virus papilloma; other conditions are erythroplasia, basal cell carcinoma, intra-epidermal carcinoma, subpreputial epithelioma.

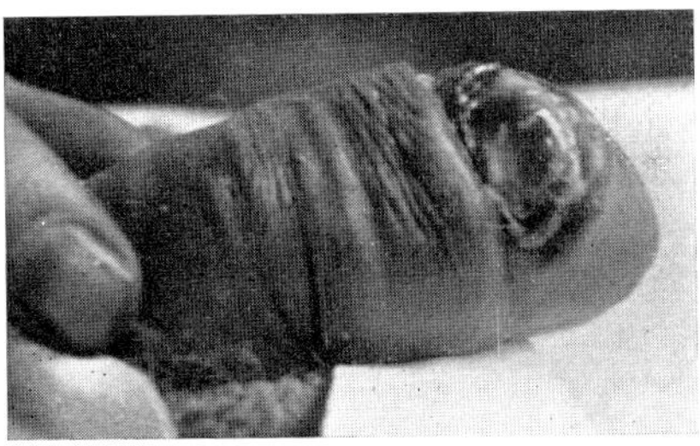

FIG. 130.

Ulcerative balanitis with early phagedena affecting glans penis. Note blackening of tissue and line of demarcation. (See also Fig. 153).

SYMPTOMS AND SIGNS

The condition is not infrequently associated with phimosis, in which case there is a further secondary infection and an exaggeration of symptoms.

There is some degree of heat, irritation or pain. Dysuria and frequency may be present. There is a thin, sometimes foul, yellow discharge beneath the prepuce, and the membrane beneath it is reddened and oedematous. Maceration, erosion or deeper ulceration may be present. The inguinal lymph nodes may be slightly enlarged and tender.

TREATMENT

This depends on the cause and the degree of inflammation. Specific causes should be treated, whether infective, traumatic, idiosyncratic or constitutional. Local therapy is best kept to bathing with normal saline or 1 : 8000 potassium permanganate in solution, and the application of a simple ointment such as zinc-and-caster oil; or in cases of irritation, allergy or eczematisation, with steroid ointment such as 1 per cent betamethasone valerate. In cases of phimosis the prepuce should be gently stretched daily after massage with lanolin or vaseline.

PHIMOSIS AND PARAPHIMOSIS

Phimosis denotes an abnormally small opening in the prepuce, preventing its retraction. Paraphimosis is the condition when such a prepuce is retracted and held tightly behind the corona glandis. Phimosis may be present at birth or result from any of the causes of preputial inflammation (p. 143). Retraction of a congenitally phimotic prepuce or one rendered phimotic by local inflammatory oedema may result in paraphimosis.

TREATMENT

Treatment of inflammatory phimosis is essentially that of the balanoposthitis (p. 144). A recent paraphimosis should be reduced by pressure on the glans, pushing steadily with both thumbs down on the glans, the paraphimotic ring being help firmly between the first and second fingers. In certain cases general anaesthesia is required.

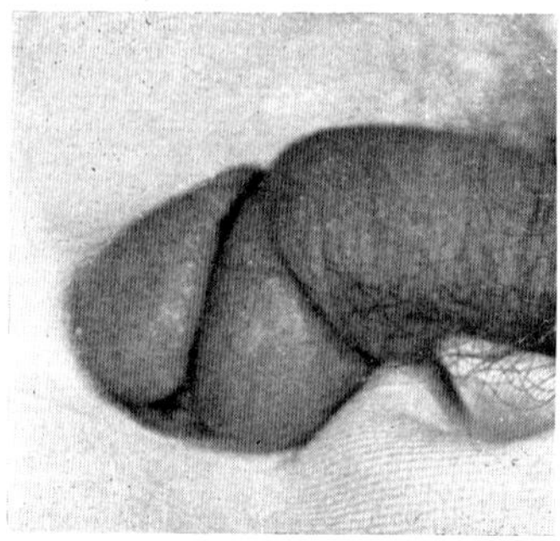

FIG. 131.
Paraphimosis.

VULVITIS, VAGINITIS AND CERVICITIS

The infective and non-infective causes of vulvitis, vaginitis and cervicitis in women are similar to those resulting in genital inflammation in the male, urethritis and balanitis. Symptoms which are mainly vulval may have as their cause a vaginal or cervical inflammation; a thorough examination should therefore never be omitted.

Thrush and trichomonas infection are common in women; non-specific vaginitis and cervicitis and erosion of cervix occur frequently. It is not clear whether or to what extent mycoplasma is involved in inflammation and transmitted infection. However, the ability of the gonococcus (*N. gonorrhoeae*) to infect and to result in complications within the female genital tract is of paramount importance (p. 125). It is of greater danger to women than to men, and the difficulties of diagnosis in women have already been stressed.

VULVITIS

Vulvitis may result from any of the conditions enumerated under causes of balanoposthitis (p. 143). Perhaps the commonest lesions are those due to the causes of intertrigo or the dermatoses (p. 172). Scabies, relatively common on the male genitalia, occurs on the thighs, abdomen and even breast in women. Vulvitis, secondary to vaginitis and cervicitis, is common, and the gonococcus, trichomonas and candida must be excluded as a routine. Infective lesions include the various conditions described earlier (Part 1) whether presenting as papules, vesicles or ulcers.

Atrophic vulvitis occurs in post-menopausal women. *Leukoplakia vulvae* is characterised by a chronic inflammation, resulting in a white appearance of the mucocutaneous epithelium. These signs slowly give place to a thin atrophic area, and may be complicated later by carcinoma. *Kraurosis vulvae* refers to atrophy of the surface epithelium with some recession of the vaginal and urethral orifices. Urethral *caruncle* is often present. Oestrogen therapy is indicated (p. 148).

Infective papilloma (vulval wart, *condyloma acuminatum*) is common. Secondary infection of this and of other neoplastic lesions may also be seen.

Vulval ulcers may result as an extension of vulvitis due to many causes. Common vesiculo-ulceration is that due to Herpes simplex progenitalis (p. 168). An acute variety of ulcer occasionally is seen, very distressing to the patient, known as *ulcus vulvae acutum* (Lipschütz): these lesions always heal in a matter of weeks and are best treated with 1 : 8000 potassium permanganate in solution, with or without betamethasone valerate ointment. This acute vulval ulceration is probably allied in its causation to buccal aphthae. One form of painful ulceration with a tendency to recurrence is due to the mucocutaneous disorder of Behçet (p. 147). Herpes Zoster or a transferred vaccinia, tuberculous or diphtheritic ulcers rarely occur.

Behçet's Syndrome

This disorder is thought to be due to an allergic vasculitis. Its main symptoms are aphthous and ulcerative lesions in the buccal and genital epithelium as well as iridocyclitis. It has a strong tendency to recurrence. In half the patients there occurs either an erythema nodosum or an acneiform rash. Malaise may be present with swelling of many of the lymph nodes. The onset of neurological signs brings with it a bad prognosis. Since genital lesions can precede those in the mouth and eyes, any erosions which develop into persisting or relapsing ulcerations should receive consideration. Local steroid therapy is less successful than that given by mouth (p. 164).

Vaginitis

The vagina's defence against bacterial infection lies primarily in the acid fluid (pH 4·5–5·0) in which its epithelium is bathed. This is maintained by action of the commensal Döderlein's bacillus (*Lactobacillus acidophilus*) which splits the glycogen present in the epithelium, through lactose, to lactic acid.

The causes of vaginitis in the adult may be summarised as:—

1. *Non-specific*

Foreign bodies and neglect of hygiene in the use of tampons, pessaries and contraceptives, douching; trauma; mixed bacterial flora of coccal and bacillary (mainly Gram-negative) type; atrophic vaginitis; vaginitis secondary to cervicitis; diabetes mellitus.

2. *Specific Infective*

This includes *T. vaginalis*, *Candida*, *mycoplasma*, and, less commonly, certain pathogenic bacteria such as *Haemophilus vaginalis*, *Staphylococcus aureus*, *Streptococcus*, *E. coli*. (*Neisseria gonorrhoeae* infects the cervix primarily, as does the *TRIC virus*).

The symptoms of discharge, dysuria, 'burning', and pain or dyspareunia may accompany many disorders of the vagina. In a young person dysuria points to an urethral or bladder infection which frequently accompanies gonorrhoea. In acute trichomonas infection pain and pruritus may be complained of; in candida irritation is the foremost symptom. When there is secondary vaginitis the Döderlein bacilli tend to disappear and hence the vaginal fluid to become less acid; the return of these bacilli after treatment is a favourable sign.

TREATMENT

The cause of vaginitis is not always clear, and may be due to several factors. Even when the aetiology is in doubt it is useful to treat the disorder with vaginal pessaries (such as stovarsol vaginal compound or penotrane), two to be inserted for two or three nights, then one nightly for a fortnight, and to instruct the patient to desist for a while from coitus, insertion of tampons or contraceptive cap, etc.

The treatment of specific vaginitis caused by the trichomonas or by candida has been discussed (p. 150). When it is thought to be due to a bacterium such as *Haemophilus*, or even *mycoplasma*, it is advisable to prescribe a wide spectrum antibiotic by mouth (tetracycline 0·25 g. six-hourly for five days), and a vaginal pessary to be inserted nightly for 10 to 14 days.

Postmenopausal vaginitis should be treated with oestrogens

either by vaginal suppository containing stilboestrol 0·5 mg. nightly for three weeks; or preferably, by small doses orally, ethinyl oestradiol 0·02–0·05 mg. daily for three weeks.

CERVICITIS

Inflammation may be acute or chronic, and involve both the endo-cervix and the vaginal cervix.

The causes of cervicitis may be:—

1. *Acute*

Usually the *N. gonorrhoeae* or *streptococci*; *Herpes simplex*; *C. oculogenitale* (TRIC virus); *Candida* and *mycoplasma* may also be isolated.

2. *Chronic*

A variety of bacteria usually in a lascerated cervix; any cause of specific infective lesion discussed in Part 1; or due to uncertain cause.

SYMPTOMS AND SIGNS

Acute purulent cervicitis occurs in gonorrhoea (p. 112) and is, less commonly, due to other causes. The virus *C. oculogenitale* results in lesions similar to those in the male urethra, occurring around the external cervical os.

Mixed bacterial and mycoplasmal infection of the cervix appears to occur in a variety of circumstances; and is common in parous women. This gives rise to urethritis, in a number of cases, in the male partner.

Herpes simplex, as a primary infection of the cervix, can cause an acute ulcerative cervicitis of some severity. The diagnosis is made by the occurrence of herpes elsewhere, and in the male partner, and also by the rise in serum antibodies to the virus (p. 168).

In the subacute and chronic stages of non-specific cervicitis there is a variety of clinical appearances: the vaginal cervix may be normal but the endocervix thickened and with a purulent secretion; the cervical os may be surrounded by a more or less granular area, or erosion; the vaginal surface of the cervix may present a few 'pointing' purulent glands or clear retention cysts; there may be eversion of the endocervical membrane.

The exclusion of a syphilitic lesion should never be neglected.

TREATMENT

The primary infective cause of the cervicitis requires treatment. An intra-uterine contraceptive device should be removed when there is more serious infection. Chronic cervicitis may be treated with wide spectrum antibiotics by mouth (for example, tetracycline 0·25 g. q.d.s. for five days) together with vaginal pessaries. Superficial erosions may slowly yield to pessaries; they may be 'touched' with 5–10 per cent silver nitrate stick, and if treated by electro-cauterisation, it is best to admit the patient to hospital.

THRUSH

Candida albicans, including other strains, is probably one of the commonest causes of vulval and vaginal symptoms, flourishing especially in pregnancy, following antibiotic therapy, and when glycosuria is present. The chief symptom is irritation, which may be severe. The discharge is usually slight and may be of whitish caseous appearance. Yellow-white patches which are slightly adherent are found on the moist areas of the vulva or vagina. The epithelial surface may be pink or raw-red. The appearance on the skin is that of an intertrigo with outlying red papules.

Under the microscope the Gram-stained vaginal smear contains epithelium, leucocytes, Döderlein bacilli with or without many secondary bacteria, and deep blue-purple staining oval yeasts or blastospores. Filaments or hyphae are less common.

TREATMENT

Antibiotic pessaries, nystatin or amphotericin, two inserted into the fornix at night for 10 to 14 nights is required. Chemical pessaries may also be used, for example Penotrane (hydrargaphen). Since one-third of patients are alimentary carriers, this state should be demonstrated if possible by faecal culture, and nystatin, 0·5 million units t.d.s., taken by mouth for 10 days in order to remove the alimentary thrush, and diminish the risk of relapse from this source. Antifungal cream or lotion (*e.g.* amphotericin) may be applied to the vulva.

TRICHOMONAS INFECTION (*T. vaginalis*)

This sexually transmitted infection is more frequently and more readily recognised in women than in men (p. 139). The inflammation, notably in young women and girls, can be acute and severe. In cases of trichomonas vaginitis there is vulval itching, burning pain and discharge. There may be dyspareunia, and the patient may complain of a dull lower abdominal ache. In acute cases the discharge is profuse, purulent and frequently malodorous.

Examination usually reveals a vulvitis. In some patients there is an accompanying intertrigo in the groin. There is a greenish-yellow, frothy discharge of high pH. The vaginal epithelium is red with desquamation over the rugae, giving rise to bleeding points and a 'strawberry' appearance. The redness and injection involves the whole vagina and vaginal cervix. The organism burrows between the cells of the vaginal epithelium. It may reach the bladder or ureters, resulting in urethritis, cystitis or pyelitis: whether it causes salpingitis is not known for certain, although an equivalent epididymitis is known to occur in men.

Whether there are extragenital sites where the protozoon may be harboured and from whence infection may be transmitted, is not known. The genital organism differs slightly from the alimentary one (*T. hominis*). The trichomonas dies more rapidly than a bacterium outside the body and in water it succumbs within the hour; cross-infection is therefore unlikely.

A low-grade subacute infection with the trichomonas is met with especially in middle life. The symptoms and signs may be minimal, and in such cases the organism may easily escape notice unless several specimens are examined.

DIAGNOSIS

This is made by wet-film and preferably by dark-ground examination of the vaginal exudate. The protozoon is 16 μ to 28 μ in length, oval in shape, with four flagella anteriorly and an undulating membrane. It may be recognised at once by its jerky movements. There are also staining methods which take longer and are not more reliable (Ch. 13). Finally it may be demonstrated by characteristic changes in the exfoliative cytology.

TREATMENT

Elimination of the trichomonas is possible in nearly all cases by the use of metronidazole 200 mg. *t.d.s.* for a week. In less than 10 per cent of women a larger dose, or more prolonged course of the drug, is required. It is more difficult however to clear up the infection during the later months of pregnancy. Trichomonicidal vaginal pessaries (*e.g.* stovarsol (acetarsol vaginal compound) or penotrane (hydrargaphen) pessaries B.N.F.) may be used concurrently in difficult cases.

SELECTED BIBLIOGRAPHY FOR NON-GONOCOCCAL INFLAMMATORY DISCHARGES AND NON-SPECIFIC URETHRITIS

General

VAGINITIS

Teokharov, B. E. (1969). *Br. J. vener. Dis.* **45,** In press.

PROSTATITIS

Oates, J. K. (1969). *Hosp. Med. No.* **2,** 556.

SYMPOSIUM ON LOWER GENITO-URINARY DISORDER (1960)

Urologia internat. **9,** no. 3–6.

Gynaecologia **149,** suppl.

Hyperimmunity

Weston, T. E. T. (1965). *Br. J. vener. Dis.* **41,** 107.

BEHÇET'S SYNDROME

Hills, E. A. (1967). *Br. med. J.* **1,** 152.

Virus–Chlamydia Oculogenitale

Dunlop, E. M. C., Al-Hussaini, M. K., Garland, J. A., Treharne, J. D., Harper, I. A. & Jones, B. R. (1965). *Lancet*, **1,** 1125, 1286.

Dunlop, E. M. C., Harper, I. A. & Al-Hussaini, M. K. (1967). *Am. J. Ophthal.* **63,** Suppl. 1073.

Holt, S., Pederson, A. M. B., Wang, S. P., Kenny, G. E., Foy, H. M. & Grayston, J. T. (1967). *Am. J. Ophthal.* **63,** 1057.

OPHTHALMIA NEONATORUM

Watson, P. G. & Gairdner, D. (1968). *Br. med. J.* **2,** 527.

Mycoplasma

Klieneberger-Nobel, E. (1962). *Mycoplasmataceae (PPLO)*. London: Academic Press.

Lancet (1967), **1,** 1044; **2,** 248.

Holt, S., Pederson, A. M. B., Wang, S. P., Kenny, G. E., Foy, H. M. & Grayston, J. T. (1967). *Am. J. Ophthal.* **63,** 1057.

Grimble, A. (1968). *Br. J. vener. Dis.* **44,** 230.

Jones, D. M. (1967). *Br. med. J.* **1,** 338.

Ludvik, W., Sachder, K. S., Flamm, M. & Seichter, I. (1967). *Wien. klin. Wschr.* **79,** 180.

T-STRAIN

Csonka, G. W., Williams, R. E. O. & Corse, J. (1966). *Lancet*, **1,** 1292.

Trichomonas Vaginalis

MEDIA

Rayner, C. F. A. (1968). *Br. J. vener. Dis.* **44,** 63.

CLINICAL: EPIDIDYMITIS

Amar, A. O. (1967). *J. Am. med. Ass.* **200,** 417.

CLINICAL: REVIEW OF THE LITERATURE

Gallai, Z. & Sylvestre, L. (1966). *Appl. Ther.* **8,** 773.

CLINICAL: TRICHOMONIASIS

Watt, L. (1965). *Practitioner*, **195,** 613.

EPIDEMIOLOGICAL AND CLINICAL: IN WOMEN

Naguib, S. M., Cornstock, G. W. & Davis, H. J. (1966). *Obstet. Gynec. N.Y.* **27,** 607.

EPIDEMIOLOGICAL AND CLINICAL: IN WOMEN AND MEN

Glebski, J. (1965). *Przegl. Derm. Wener.* **52,** 617.

EPIDEMIOLOGICAL AND CLINICAL: IN MEN

De Luca, M., & Argenziano, G. (1965). *Dermatatologia, Napoli*, **15,** 339.

Candida

GENITAL AND ANORECTAL

Rohatiner, J. J. (1966). *Br. J. vener. Dis.* **42,** 197.

'Squibb' Symposium (1966). London.

FLUORESCENT ANTIBODY TEST

Rohatiner, J. J. & Grimble, A. (1967). *J. Obstet. Gynec. Br. Commonw.* **74,** 875.

Bacterial

Furneso, G. & Csonka, G. W. (1966). *Br. J. vener. Dis.* **42,** 185.

Symposium (1960) Urologia internat., and Gynaecologia.

CHAPTER 9

Genito-Urinary Rheumatism and the Polyarthritic Syndrome (Brodie, Fiessinger-Leroy or Reiter's syndrome)

INTRODUCTION

This syndrome is characterised by an abacterial urethritis, conjunctivitis, and arthritis which is usually polyarticular. No causal agent has yet been identified to account for all cases; and, as with most other forms of rheumatism, the precise mechanism producing the disorder is obscure. The condition was described by Brodie and others in the last century and more recently by Leroy and Fiessinger, and Reiter.

A similar polyarthritis occurs in bacterial dysentery and in other alimentary disorders. This syndrome also has been described for many years in untreated gonorrhoea. Arthritis and rheumatism when they occur in gonorrhoea are thought to be due, in this country at the present time, to the same cause as a rheumatism resulting from non-gonococcal genital inflammation. But there is no proof that gonorrhoea itself does not result in a polyarthritic syndrome, as described in the days before specific treatment existed. In neither case does the genital inflammation respond entirely to antibiotic or chemotherapy. But in gonococcal urethritis the *N. gonorrhoeae* disappears from the exudate along with the specific treatment.

The complete syndrome is relatively rare. An isolated example of rheumatism, however, such as arthralgia, arthritis of short duration, soft tissue rheumatism, conjunctivitis, circinate balanitis or, less frequently, iritis, is not uncommon with lower genito-urinary infection in men. The incidence of minor attacks is probably higher than 3–4 per cent which is the usual incidence for the more severe ones. The disorder is at least 10 times commoner in men than in women.

CLINICAL FEATURES

The onset is with an abacterial urethritis, which varies greatly in severity, and usually has an incubation period of one to three weeks. Generally there is a first-glass urinary haze, or a first glass of urine containing flakes or small threads. Evidence of prostato-vesiculitis is almost always present. However, the acuteness of the genito-urinary signs bears *no* relationship to the severity of the disease.

A week or more after the appearance of the discharge a conjunctivitis and episcleritis arise, unilaterally then bilaterally. In some cases conjunctivitis is absent or fleeting. On the other hand it is not uncommon for conjunctivitis to occur alone as a complication of urethritis in men. Where there are recurrent exacerbations of the conjunctivitis the course of the concomitant arthritis also tends to be capricious.

The onset of arthritis, often heralded by pain, occurs during the second or third week. The disease however may be mainly arthralgic with only pains in the joints. Polyarthritis is commoner than monarticular arthritis. It develops rapidly, not symmetrically as a rule, the number of joints involved reaching a maximum early in the attack. There is swelling of the joints due to synovitis, along with pain and restriction of movements. The joints are also to some degree hot and tender. The larger joints take longer to clear up than the smaller ones, residual swelling being due to capsular thickening and pericapsular infiltration.

There is a characteristic distribution of joint damage in this syndrome, joints of the lower limbs being involved more frequently than those of the upper, and peripheral joints more often than central (*i.e.*, hip and shoulder girdle). Acromioclavicular, sternoclavicular or temperomandibular arthritis is more likely to be noted in this than in other joint disorders.

Sacro-iliitis is not uncommonly present. Spinal lesions, however, are rare.

At the beginning of the attack, the patient complains of malaise. There is usually intermittent and irregular pyrexia, sometimes returning to normal within a matter of days, at times remaining unsettled for one to three months. The E.S.R. is

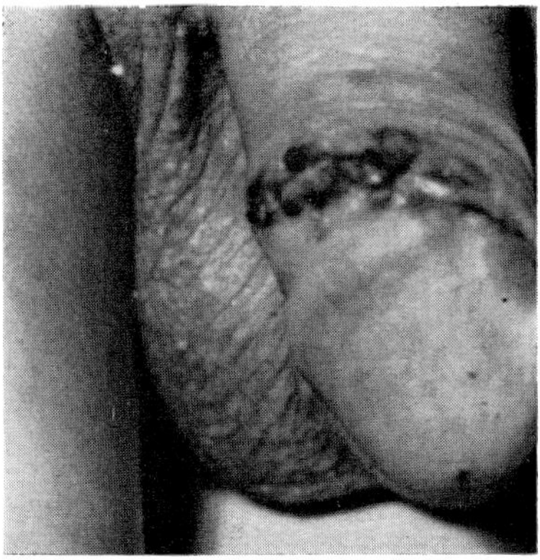

FIG. 132.
Keratodermia blenorrhagica: crusting lesions of prepuce.

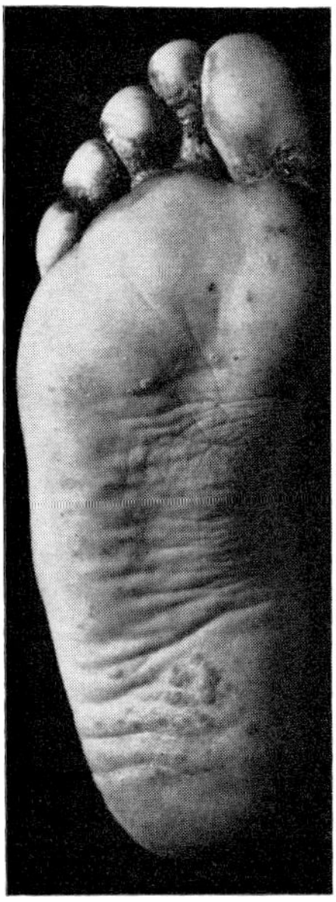

FIG. 133*a*.

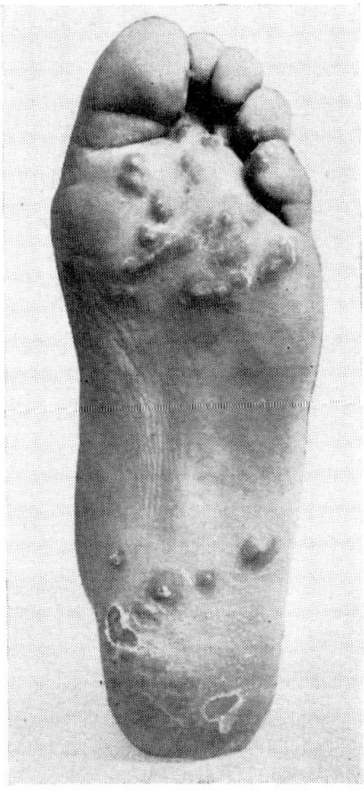

FIG. 133*b*.

Keratodermia blenorrhagica: papulo-nodular lesions of soles of feet

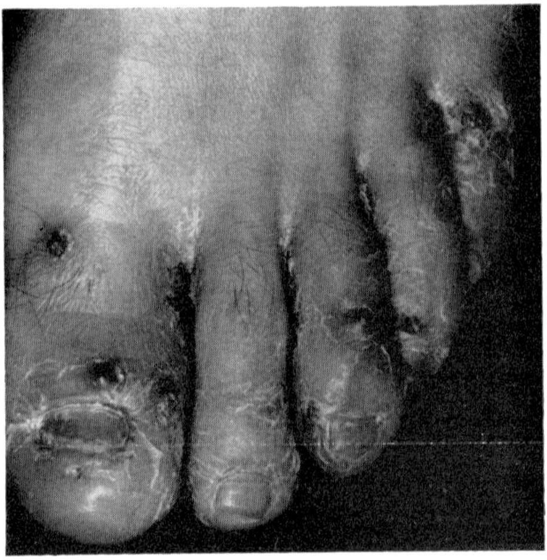

FIG. 134.
Keratodermia blenorrhagica: papulo-nodular lesions of toes and nails.

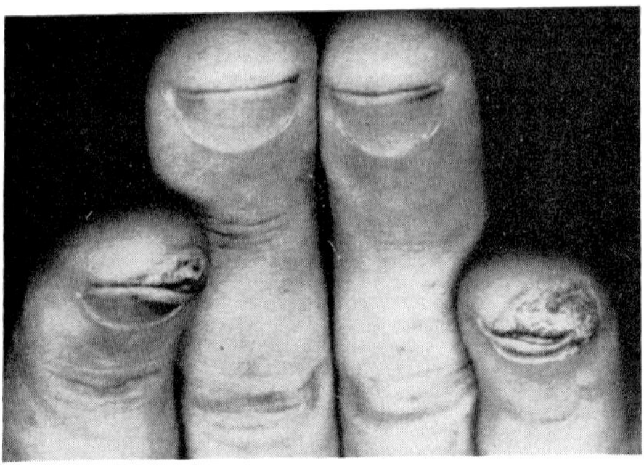

FIG. 135.
Keratodermia blenorrhagica: lesions of the nails of the fingers.

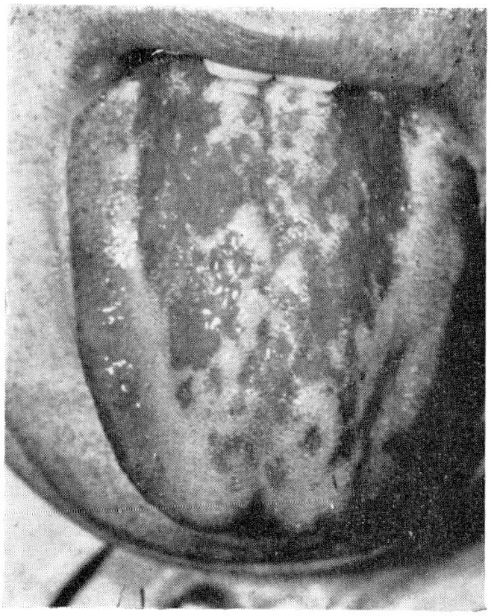

FIG. 136.
Erosions of the tongue.

raised during the periods of active disease, perhaps greatly so (over 100 mm. in the first hour). Marked loss of weight may follow

Along with the urethritis there occur mucocutaneous manifestations. Of these *balanitis circinata* is the commonest, presenting as shallow pink erosions with raised white edges, coalescing and forming circinate outlines. In the circumcised patient the selesions may be scaly. Skin lesions, known as *kerotadermia blennorrhagica*, may be noted in a tenth to a quarter of all cases, the commonest site for their occurrence being the soles of the feet. The condition is seen after the first two weeks, beginning with vesicles or 'pustules'. Keratinisation takes place and the resulting lesions are either soft and limpet-like, or firm, parakeratotic and nodular. They have to be distinguished in particular from rupial syphilides and psoriasis.

Changes in the *nails* include involvement of the nail fold and cellular accumulation beneath the nail plate, which becomes yellow, thickened, and then lifts.

Stomatitis is the least common of the mucocutaneous signs, and appears as vesicles and superficial ulcers involving any part of the mouth, tongue or inside of the lips.

Inflammation may occur in many of the tissues of the locomotor system: for example perichondritis, especially of the rib cartilage; tendonitis and tenosynovitis, or bursitis, appear as painful swellings close to the bony insertions, particularly the Achilles tendons and bursae.

Plantar fascitis is a common and important sign and always suggests the diagnosis of the disease. The sole of the foot especially in front of the heel is painful, tender, and at times swollen and red. A particular deformity of the feet (equivalent to the ulnar deviation of the hand in a rheumatoid patient) is unique to this disorder.

Conjunctivitis occurs frequently and early in the disease. In a number of patients, however, whose attacks are severe and long lasting, or who suffer from repeated attacks, *iritis* (anterior non-granular uveitis) becomes increasingly prominent. It may be on one or both sides, or alternate. Repeated affection of the same eye may lead to serious damage. In a few patients the recurrent attacks are dominated by the eye lesion. The not uncommon association of iritis, without arthritis, in men with lower genito-urinary inflammation must be remembered.

In rare cases *visceral* involvement is more extensive. Lymphadenitis, thrombophlebitis, cardiac lesions which include pericarditis, endocarditis and aortic incompetence, a dry pleurisy, or symptoms and signs in the central nervous system may be noted.

Radiological changes are usually absent in the acute phase. Early changes consist of: patchy osteoporosis adjacent to affected joints; and later 'erosions' or small points of bony destruction usually at the periphery of the articular surface (especially to be seen in the os calcis). Later, chronic changes may be noted such as: periostitis, which, together with erosions, is common at the base of the os calcis; sacro-iliitis in the shape of marginal irregularities and sclerosis; and chronic arthritis where, after failure to resolve, there occurs new bone formation and sclerosis, loss of joint space, destruction and occasionally ankylosis. These changes are more likely to be seen in the feet than elsewhere. A diagnosis of Reiter's syndrome from the X-rays is made more on the distribution of the changes than by any single characteristic one. The appearance of the os calcis with erosions and periostitis is however near diagnostic; yet similar changes may occasionally be seen in ankylosing spondylitis.

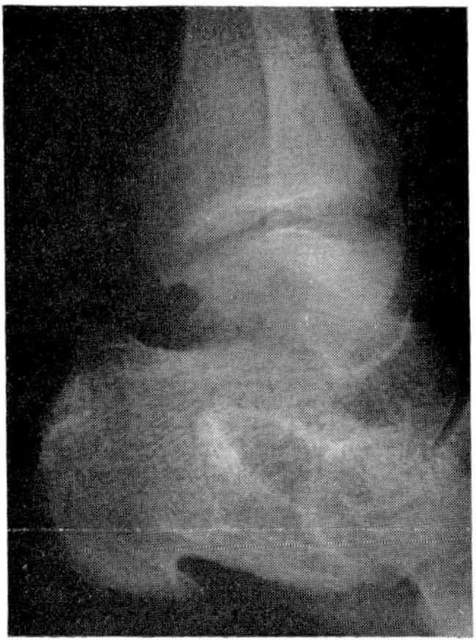

FIG. 137.

Calcaneal 'spur'.

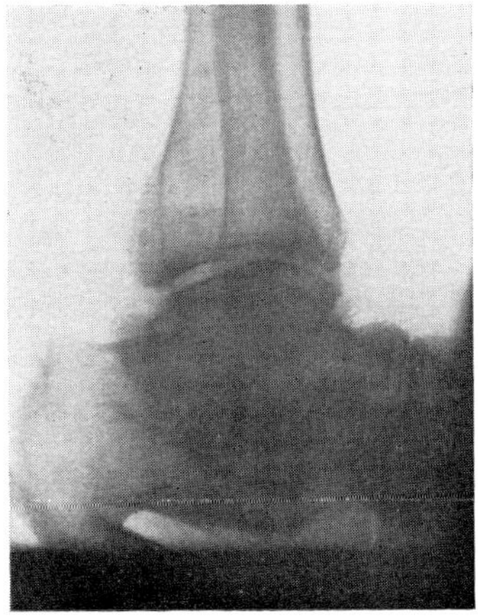

FIG. 138.

Osteoperiostial reaction at the lower end of the tibia and the calcaneum; the mid-tarsal joint is also involved.

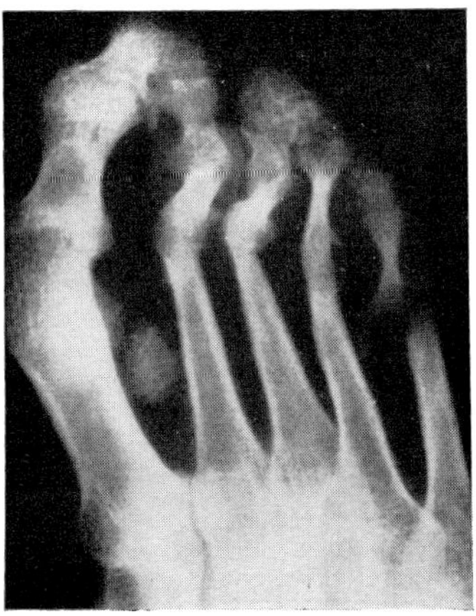

FIG. 139.

Fibular-deviation' deformity of the toes with destruction of interphalangeal joints.

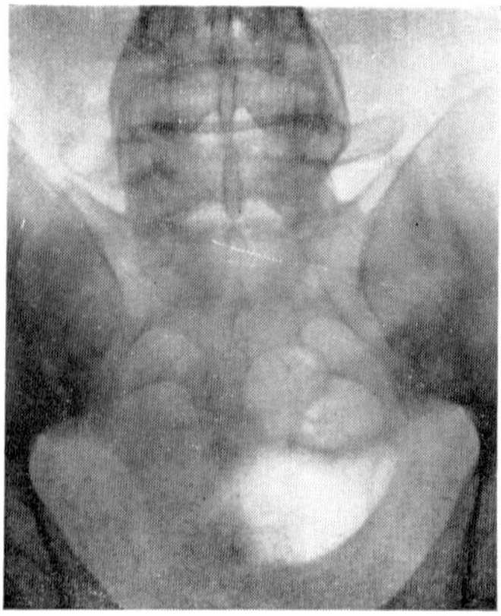

FIG. 140.

Sacro-ileitis and advanced lumbar spondylitis.

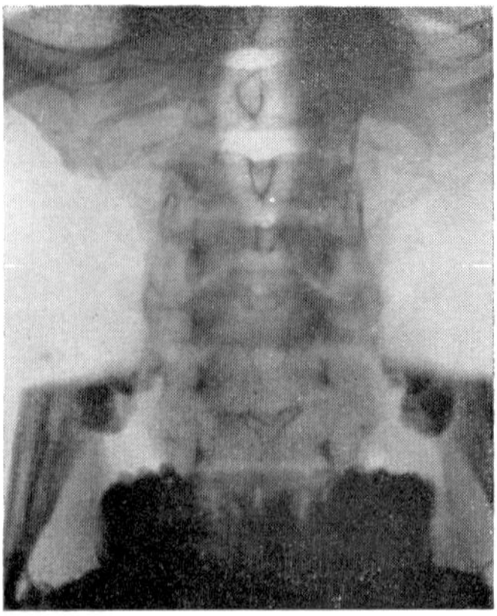

FIG. 141.

Cervical vertebrae, showing ankylosing spondylitic changes in a patient with chronic Reiter's syndrome.

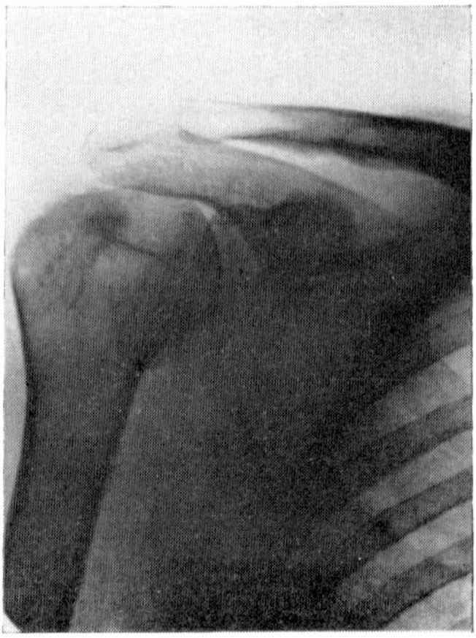

FIG. 142.

Osteoperiostitis of the head of humerus, in the region of the greater tubercle.

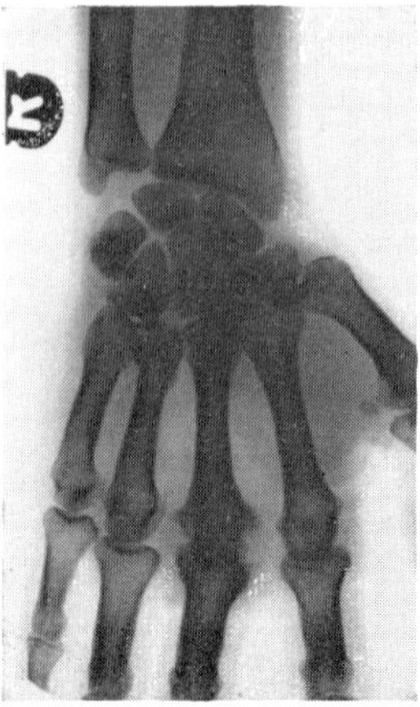

FIG. 143.

Severe arthritis of metatarso-phalangeal joints in chronic Reiter's syndrome, showing 'punched-out' areas in juxta-articular bone with osteophytic outgrowth, seen also in rheumatoid arthritis and similar disorders.

LABORATORY CRITERIA

Apart from a raised E.S.R., there may be a mild anaemia (hypochromic or microcytic) and a slight polymorphonuclear leucocytosis in the active stages of the disease.

Serum protein changes occur in the most severe cases, resulting in an increase in globulin, usually IgA, less commonly IgG. The rheumatoid factor is absent. The synovial exudate contains at first polymorphonuclear leucocytes and later a greater proportion of lymphocytes. No unanimity yet exists concerning the significance of various micro-organisms grown from tissue or from synovial exudate: these include a virus, mycoplasma and occasionally bacteria. Usually the joint fluid (bacteriologically) is sterile. An auto-allergy to prostatic tissue has been demonstrated in male patients. The roles of mycoplasma and the TRIC virus as possible aetiological agents are uncertain.

DIFFERENTIAL DIAGNOSIS

When the disorder presents with the classical triad: *urethritis*, *conjunctivitis* and *arthritis*, the diagnosis is straightforward. Should the condition be seen, however, with only one of the main features or any of the other less common individual symptoms and signs, difficulties arise.

In particular, cases of conjunctivitis and uveitis in men should be examined for inflammation in the lower genito-urinary tract, especially of the prostate; and other signs of rheumatism must be looked for.

Similarly, in all cases of rheumatism and arthritis in men it behoves one to exclude genito-urinary infection with prostatitis, since cases of Reiter's syndrome may present atypically, either with an ocular lesion, or as monoarticular arthritis or soft-tissue rheumatism.

Many of the features of Reiter's syndrome overlap those of the more common arthritic disorders.

Rheumatoid arthritis begins more often with a period of malaise, progressing to a polyarthritis involving first the small joints of the hands: when this disorder is atypical and starts for example as a monoarticular arthritis in the lower limbs the diagnosis is more difficult. The Latex (rheumatoid) test is positive after a few months.

The onset of ankylosing spondylitis is usually with a persisting backache, the central and vertebral joints being involved first. Sacro-iliitis and calcaneal periostitis occur both in this disorder and in Reiter's syndrome and the appearance of certain cases may be very alike. But Reiter's syndrome hardly ever affects the spine to any degree.

Psoriasis (in which the skin lesions can be very similar to those of keratodermia blennorrhagica) and bacillary dysentery give rise to arthropathies almost indistinguishable from Reiter's syndrome. Other alimentary tract disorders may cause arthritis: regional enteritis and ulcerative colitis. Other so-called muco-cutaneous syndromes may, rarely, cause arthritis; Stevens-Johnson syndrome and Behçet's syndrome; also drug and serum reactions, and erythema nodosum.

Rheumatic fever begins with a more flitting type of arthritis, follows a sore throat due to an α-haemolytic streptococcus, and has a much higher incidence of cardiac symptoms or renal involvement. Lupus erythematosus (disseminated), which is due to an immunological disorder, may result in arthritis, usually involving the hands.

Other causes of arthritis which should be excluded are: infective, gonococcal, tubercular, rarely syphilitic, brucellosis, typhoid, and all other causes of bacteriaemia; gout, where there is accompanying hyperuricaemia; and traumatic.

COURSE AND PROGNOSIS

In the very mild form of rheumatism the patient may have a genital infection, evidence of prostatitis, a minimal arthritis or conjunctivitis and little general reaction. Many such cases may escape diagnosis.

The average duration of an attack of the disease which is severe enough to force the patient into bed, is over three months. The severer attacks may continue in varying intensity for a year or two. It is extremely difficult to judge the duration of the disease in any individual case. Although the severe forms of the complete syndrome tend to last longer, mild attacks do not necessarily clear up quickly. The individual attacks, however, are self-limiting in the majority of cases.

Over half the patients have more than one attack, the symptom-free periods varying from a matter of months to half a life-time. The disease is recurrent and progressive in a few cases. Crippling arthritis or damage to sight from the disease is very uncommon. Death from the disease has occurred only in the isolated case.

TREATMENT

Although helpful in ameliorating certain features, specific forms of treatment appear to have a disappointing effect on the overall course the disease takes.

Treatment measures consist of (1) treatment of urethritis and prostatitis; (2) bed-rest and attention to general health and nursing care; (3) treatment of the rheumatism.

Local treatment of the prostatitis and urethritis has been described (p. 121); its duration may be extended. The patient should remain in bed as long as the temperature is raised and the E.S.R. stays high; but, unless the attack is a severe one, the patient should remain partly ambulant, getting up for toilet, etc. It is important that the joints, though rested, be kept mobile, and the muscles be exercised and kept in trim, especially those muscles serving the affected joints. This is done by passive and active joint movement, isometric muscle exercises, and physiotherapy. Aspiration of a tensely swollen joint and subsequent tight bandaging may bring relief.

The drugs of particular use in this form of rheumatism are:—acetylsalicylic acid (2·0 g. *t.d.s.*); phenylbutazone (100 mg. q.d.s. dropping to *b.d.*); indomethacin (25 mg. *q.d.s.* dropping to *b.d.* by mouth, or as suppositories). Apart from aspirin, paracetamol (0·5 g. four-hourly) or mefenamic acid (0·25 g. *q.d.s.*) may be given. Pain in the acute stage may be severe.

Corticosteroid preparations should be reserved for use in the severe attack in which the patient is very ill, or has lost a great deal of weight, and when the mucocutaneous and arthritic features of the disease are distressing. The patient should be free from hypertension, nephritis, peptic ulcer, diabetes mellitus or chronic infection such as tuberculosis. Prednisolone is given by mouth, 10 mg. *q.d.s.*, later dropping by 5 mg. every second or third day. The drug should always be 'tailed off', not withdrawn suddenly. Corticosteroids may either be used in this way for short courses in cases where improvement is very slow or has temporarily stopped; or they may be given in lower dosage (*e.g.*, prednisolone 10–20 mg. daily) for longer periods.

Nevertheless there is a more definite place for the local use of steroids. In plantar fasciitis, when walking becomes difficult or impossible, injections into the fascia or into the region of the periosteum on the anterior aspect of the calcaneum, is beneficial. Similarly, injections into the joint spaces or capsule, bursae or tendon sheaths involved in subacute or chronic stages of the disease achieve good results: prednisolone butylacetate 25 mg./ml., 1–2 ml.

SELECTED BIBLIOGRAPHY FOR GENITO-URINARY RHEUMATISM AND THE POLYARTHRITIC SYNDROME

Genito-urinary Rheumatism

RELATIONSHIP TO GENITO-URINARY INFECTION

Ford, D. K. & Rasmussen, G. (1964). *Arthritis Rheum.* **7,** 220.

REVIEW (IN ENGLISH) OF 260 CASES

Csonka, G. W. (1965). *Ergeben Lun. med. Kinderheilk.* **23,** 125.

ENDOCARDITIS

Déchelotte, J. (1966). *Cour & med. interne*, **5,** 81.

SYNOVIAL FLUID

Pekin, T. J., Malinin, T. I. & Zvaiffer, N. J. (1967). *Ann. intern. Med.* **66,** 677.

VIRUS ISOLATIONS (*Bedsoniae*)

Schachter, J. *et al.* (1966). *Proc. Soc. exp. Biol. Med.* **122,** 283.

SPONDYLITIS, ANKYLOSING

Good, A. E. (1965). *Acta rheum. scand.* **11,** 305.

NEUROLOGICAL

Catterall, R. D., Rooney, K. J. & Kirby, B. (1965). *Br. J. vener. Dis.* **41,** 62.

IN CHILDREN

Moss, I. (1964). *Br. J. vener. Dis.* **40,** 166.

TREATMENT

Wright, V. (1965). *Rheumatism*, **21,** 30.

Bernard, J. G., Badrouillard, R., Feline, A. & Lucaes, R. (1964). *Sem. Hôp. Paris*, **40,** 1935.

Part 3

Non-Venereal Disorders

CHAPTER 10

Non-Venereal Disorders of the Genitalia and their Venereal Forms Non-Syphilitic Treponematoses

Non-venereal lesions of the genitalia include a number of disorders presenting diagnostic problems, from time to time, when they have to be distinguished from venereal diseases. Several of these are sexually transmitted. They may be grouped as:—

1. Infections of the skin—such as papilloma, molluscum contagiosum, herpes simplex (rarely Zoster or vaccinia); furunculosis, impetigo, scabies, phthiriasis.
2. Dermatoses—such as psoriasis, lichen planus, pityriasis, contact dermatitis, eczemas, granuloma annulare.
3. Non-infective lesions and ulcerations—such as erythroplasia, balanitis xerotica obliterans, kraurosis vulvae, ulcus vulvae acutum, Fordyce condition, hirsuties papillaris penis, Stevens-Johnson syndrome.
4. Neoplasia.

1. Infections of the Skin

Infection due to viruses, bacteria or infestation with mites are common. *Herpes simplex* tends to cause recurrent lesions on the genitalia as often as elsewhere. Following coitus, tiny grouped vesicles appear within a week or so on keratinized or non-keratinized epithelium, especially of the glans, prepuce or vulva and sometimes cervix. They rapidly ulcerate, each showing a bright red areola. The shallow ulcers tend to coalesce and to become secondarily infected. Initially there is itching, to be followed by pain. The local lymph nodes are usually slightly enlarged during the stage of erosion. Healing occurs in about two weeks. Virus inclusions can be seen by suitable staining of vesicle contents or the organism can be grown on developing chick embryo. Primary infection can result in a more extensive ulceration, which, on the cervix, presents as a severe papulo-necrotic lesion. Serum antibody titres can be shown to rise during the attack. In secondarily infected cases, local bathes with 1 : 8000 potassium permanganate and long-acting sulphonamide 1·0 g. daily by mouth for a few days, are advisable. Local hourly application of idoxyuridine cuts short the attack.

Condyloma acuminatum (virus papilloma or wart) may occur on any part of the genitalia. There is evidence that the virus is related to that infecting general body areas and is therefore not strictly venereal. The incubation period extends to several months In the moist areas of the genitalia the lesions may assume larger cauliflower-like masses, especially in company with inflammatory conditions such as gonorrhoea. Surface erosion of the lesions results in an unpleasant secondary infection. Peri-anal masses suggest that the patient might be a passive homosexual.

Treatment of the lesions on non-keratinised epithelium is by local application of 25 per cent podophyllin in methanol. Precautions should be taken against contaminating other parts since the substance is very irritant. Application should be every three days until the lesions regress. If the wart is on the cervix it can be touched with a silver nitrate stick; those on the skin require removal with cautery or carbon dioxide snow.

Molluscum contagiosum, also due to a virus, appears as a pale papule with a typical central depression. Lesions may be multiple and occur anywhere on the skin surface. The contents of the papule if suitably stained show virus inclusions in characteristic 'balloon' cells. The papules may be treated by cautery, by a drop of phenol on a pointed stick, or by freezing with carbon dioxide snow.

Bacterial infection of the genital skin is not uncommon. Folliculitis, furunculosis or deeper pyogenic infections, usually due to the staphylococcus, occur typically in relation to hair follicles of the anogenital region. Impetigo is less common. Hidroadenitis, a recurrent pyogenc infection of the apocrine glands, occurs in the axillae but also in the anogenital area, manifesting itself as red nodules slowly eroding to the surface. These should be treated with erythromycin or tetracycline in full dosage by mouth.

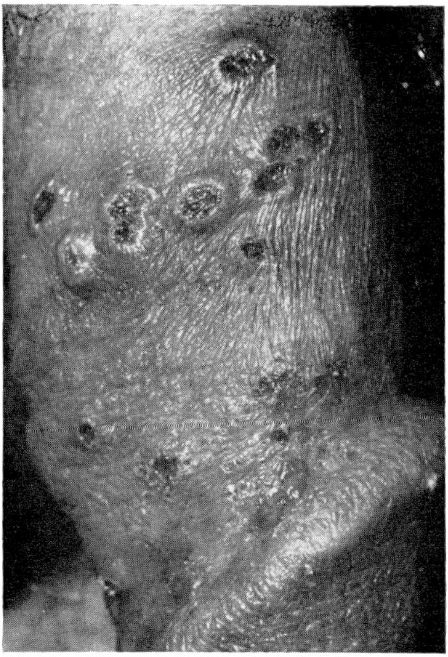

Fig. 144.
Herpes simplex of penis.

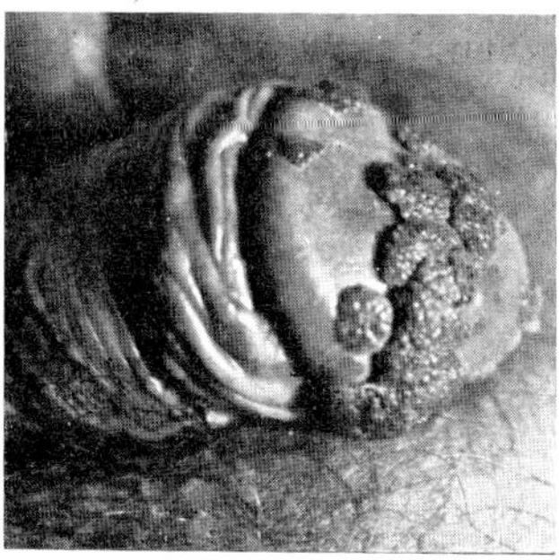

Fig. 145.
Penile warts in male.

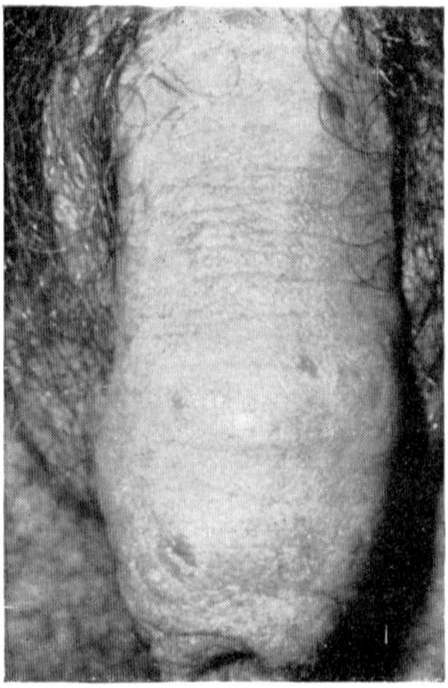

FIG. 146.

Scabies; showing the small excoriated lesions, which become more papular on the penis.

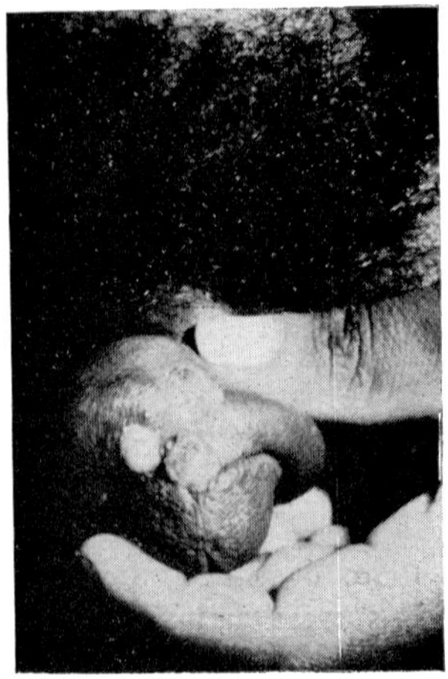

FIG. 147

'Norwegian' scabies.

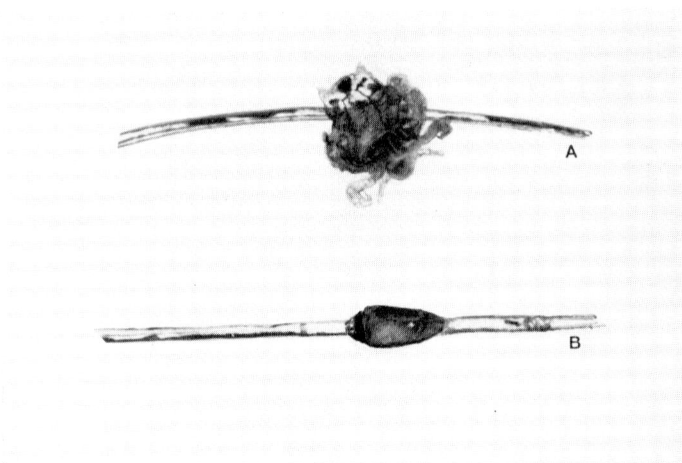

148*a*, *b* Phthyrius pubis and nit on human hairs.

Various *dermatomycoses* of the inguinal folds and anogenital region enter into the differential diagnosis of dermatitis, candidasis, psoriasis and the syphilides.

Scabies, due to *Sarcoptes scabei*, is often transmitted sexually, the lesions then being distributed on the genitalia and neighbouring areas of skin. Characteristically there is nocturnal irritation, and the appearance of small groups of papules together with greyish burrows and excoriations due to scratching. In men the lesions on the genitalia occur on the glans, prepuce and shaft of the penis. They are seen comparatively uncommonly on the genitalia in women, in whom they appear on the abdomen and thighs.

The disorder is treated by applying 25 per cent benzyl benzoate lotion over the entire body surface up to the chin for three days in succession, the patient being advised not to take a bath until treatment has been completed.

Phthirius pubis, or the crab louse, settles on the hairy parts of the anogenital region for preference. The chief symptom is irritation, increasing as the parasites multiply. They are seen firmly clinging, by the legs of only one side, to the hairs on which the eggs or nits are cemented. Greyish macules may be present in the skin where the louse has been feeding, and must be distinguished from a syphilitic roseola. A number of drugs can be used for treatment, for example, Lorexane lotion diluted 1 : 4.

2. Dermatoses

Many skin diseases involve the genitalia and have to be considered when a lesion exists in a 'venereal' context. *Psoriasis* not infrequently causes the male patient to seek venereological advice. The condition varies from a small, red lesion with silvery scales, to large, chronic, circumscribed patches which, when scraped, yield the typical bleeding points. On the prepuce the condition may occur without scaling, and in a moist area the lesions may have the appearance of a non-scaling intertrigo.

Lichen planus is characterised by the small flat-topped polygonal-shaped papula of slightly purplish hue. Whitish areas are noted in a moist lesion on the mouth or the genitalia. Itching is a prominent feature.

Contact dermatitis may present as an acute eczema with oedema, vesiculation and crusting; or with dryness, scaling and lichenification of the glans and penile or vulval skin. More frequent causes of this lesion are contraceptive chemicals and sheaths, antiseptics such as Dettol used in the bath, or medicated soaps. Similar consideration must be given to seborrhoeic dermatitis with its greasy scales, and to intertrigo. Intertrigo of the anogenital region is common, progressing from a moist erythema to fissuring and secondary infection. It is important to rid the lesions of skin bacteria, fungus or yeasts, and then treat the condition with dusting powders and a change to lighter clothing.

3. Non-Infective Lesions and Ulcerations

Erythroplasia develops as a raised, flat, velvety red patch involving the glans or coronal sulcus, less frequently the prepuce, and rarely the shaft of the penis. The lesion increases very slowly in size, the affected area of skin remaining pliable unless superficial erosion or malignant transformation takes place: how often the latter occurs is uncertain. The condition must be distinguished from eczema, lupus, intraepidermal carcinoma and syphilis.

Balanitis xerotica obliterans is a chronic, sclerotic and atrophic process involving the glans, inner surface of the prepuce and distal urethra. It is closely related to, if not identical with, kraurosis vulvae (p. 146), in women and lichen sclerosus et atrophicus. The condition is not rare and occurs as white atrophic plaques on the glans, prepuce or urethral meatus. Stenosis of the urethral orifice results. Transformation to carcinoma is rare. The topical application of steroid cream may result in a slow regression of the lesions. Circumcision is usually advised, along with dilatation of the meatus.

Non-venereal ulcerations due to various forms of bacterial infection, such as cutaneous diphtheria and papulo-necrotic tuberculide, are rare today. Ulcus vulvae acutum (Lipschütz) is a form of ulceration to be seen in young women. The aetiology is uncertain but may be allied to that of buccal aphthae (p. 147). It has to be distinguished, in particular, from herpes simplex.

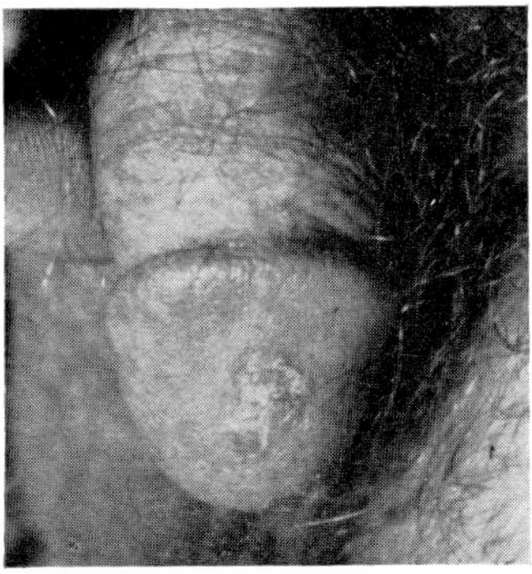

FIG. 149.

Psoriasis of the glans.

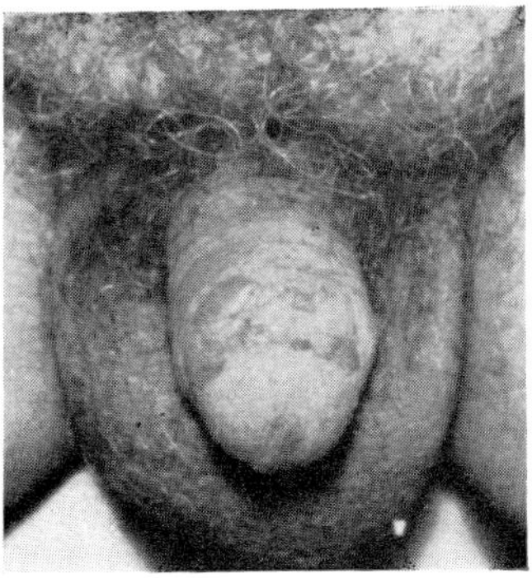

FIG. 150.

Raised pink plaques of erythroplasia.

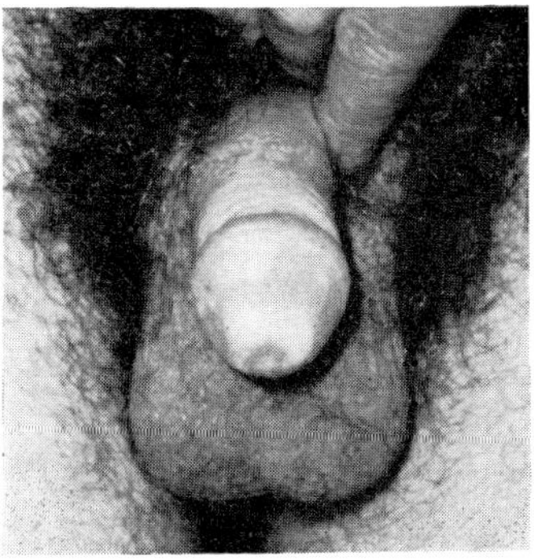

FIG. 151.

Balanitis xerotica obliterans.

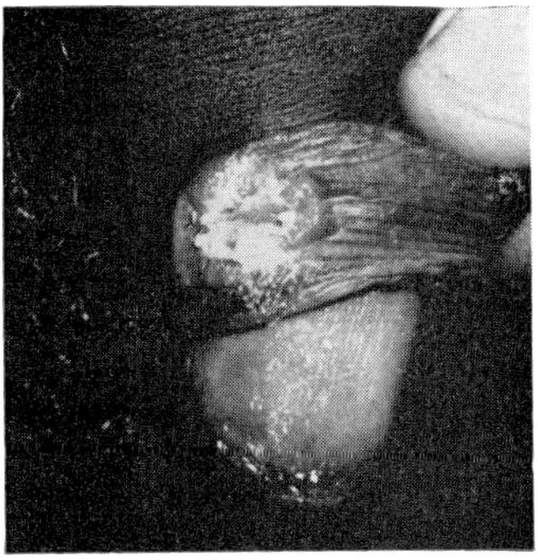

FIG. 152.

Indolent bacterial ulceration with thickening in walls, suggesting chancre: lymphadenitis present.

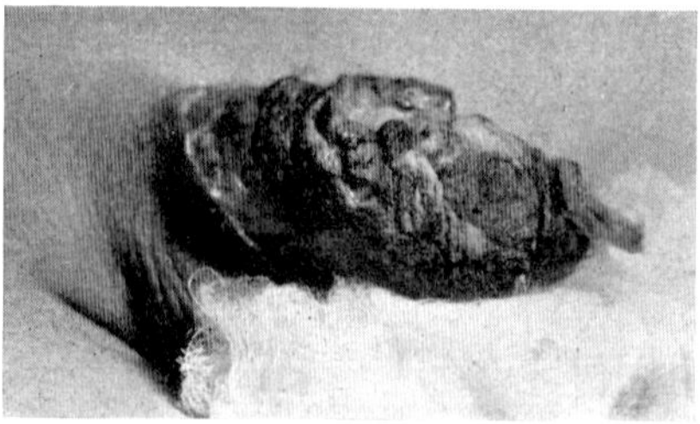

FIG. 153.

Phagedena involving integument of penis—line of demarcation immediately distal to pubes.

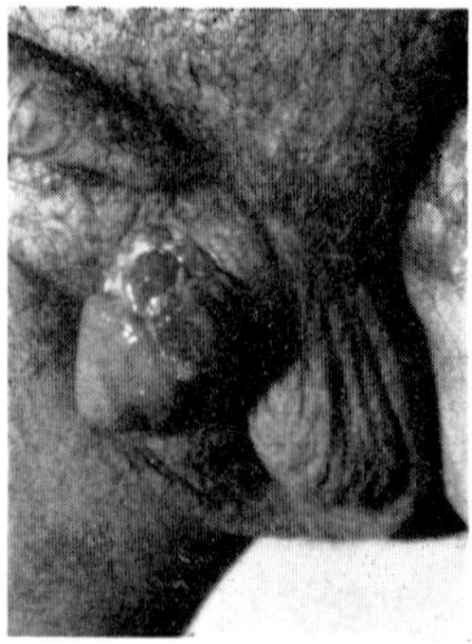

FIG. 154.

Epithelioma of corneal sulcus; raised warty appearance.

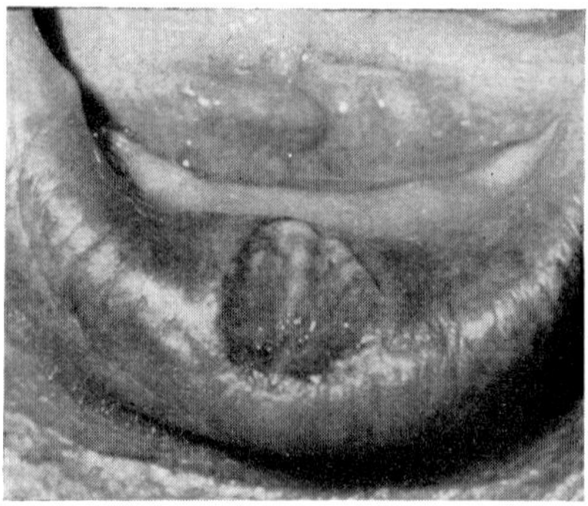

FIG. 155.

Carcinoma of lip, simulating chancre.

Ulcus gangrenosum or gangrenous changes in any penile or vulval ulceration may be induced by bacterial and fusiform organism infection in an existing traumatic or specific ulcer. The brown-green pseudomembrane and serous exudate, the rapidly increasing size of the lesion, and the foul odour should indicate the serious nature of the condition.

The lesions of erythema multiforme exudativum, *Stevens-Johnson syndrome*, consist of apthous ulceration in the mouth and moist genital epithelium, an acute ulceromembranous conjunctivitis, and papulovesicular lesions of the genitalia and extremities, rarely of the face. The cutaneous manifestations are not always present. The condition begins with moderate fever and may be accompanied by lymphocytosis; a pneumonitis may also develop. Usually the disorder clears up in a few weeks, and has a fair prognosis. Complications in the eye are uncommon. The condition sometimes follows drug treatment (especially with the sulphonamides). Treatment is by the use of antibiotics, with steroid therapy in the more severe cases.

Hirsuites papillaris penis develops in adulthood on the corona of the glans penis or glans itself, appearing as tiny elevations. They have no functional role, being residua from our animal ancestry, and show the normal histological appearance for glans epithelium.

Other causes of vulvitis and balanoposthitis (p. 143). *Behçet's* syndrome (p. 147).

4. External Neoplasms of the Genitalia

Benign cutaneous neoplasms are to be seen on the genitalia from time to time, and for a description of them reference should be made to textbooks on the subject. The commonest lesion is the virus papilloma or wart. Similarly, various malignant neoplasms may be seen. Some of these occur principally on the penis or vulva, forming lesions which have to be differentiated from those resulting from venereal disorders. Erythroplasia as a premalignant lesion has been described.

Intra-epidermal carcinoma (Bowen's) is rare on the genitalia. *Basal cell epithelioma* is occasionally seen being a warty lesion to start with, and possessing a tendency to show central ulceration.

Squamous cell carcinoma is not uncommon. It presents as a rule in the uncircumcised male, usually on the glans or prepuce, as a minute, scaly nodule or tiny ulcer. It develops slowly, becoming either more papilliferous or increasingly infiltrating. An ulcerative type also occurs. Spread is slow and via the lymphatics; but finally haematogenous metastases may occur.

Induratio Penis Plastica (Peyronie)

This condition (allied to Dupuytren's contracture in the hand) occurs as a hard thickening in the tunica albuginea of the corpora cavernosa, which in severe cases results in a bending or distortion of the organ on erection.

Priapism

Usually referred to in men (but also occurring in women in the clitoris) as a persistent, severely painful erection of the penis unaccompanied by sexual desire. It is due to stasis or thrombosis in the cavernous tissue due to such causes as injury, reticuloses, neoplasia, or to central nervous system disorder with paraplegia. Intermittent priapism can result from irritation in the posterior urethra, prostate or vesicles.

Impotence

Male sexual potency depends amongst other things upon a balanced endocrine function, being disturbed by a wide variety of endocrine disorders. Also it is disturbed by disharmony in the psyche: by tension, anxiety and depression. In the male, sexual potency most nearly follows the pattern of ketosteroid secretion, is near its greatest a few years after puberty, and begins to decline from the age of 35 years. Impotence starts to increase in the male from about this age.

Impotence, therefore, which is not physiological and part of the ageing process of the individual, is largely due to psychological causes of which the patient is or is not aware. Moreover the onset of any degree of impotence often brings with it anxieties which perpetuate and increase the malfunction. Drugs which relieve tension, anxiety and depression are thus more useful therapeutically than, for example, testosterone which has little effect in this situation.

Other causes of impotence are: (1) congenital, (2) endocrine abnormalities, (3) ill-health due to serious or chronic disease, (4) diseases of the central nervous system affecting the sexual mechanism.

NON-SYPHILITIC TREPONEMATOSES

The pathogenic *treponema*, a subspecies of the *spirochaeticae*, is very common throughout the world. There are many non-syphilitic strains which are morphologically indistinguishable from the *T. pallidum* of syphilis, and furthermore, these strains stimulate the formation of antibodies which up to the present cannot satisfactorily be distinguished from syphilitic antibodies.

The non-syphilitic treponemes differ slightly in their infectivity of man and certain laboratory animals*, and it is largely in the clinical manifestations and mode of spread (non-sexually) that the diagnostic differences lie.

It would appear that the non-syphilitic treponemes are very nearly allied since there are many similarities in the diseases caused by them, and it is significant that these diseases on the whole exist in different areas of the world. However they all occur in the tropical and subtropical regions and are spread by non-sexual means.

Yaws (*T. pertenue*) exists widely throughout the warmer regions, especially those having a high rainfall. Bejel (*T.* of Bejel) exists among the Arabs, particularly in the Euphrates valley, and an identical disease is to be seen in parts of Africa. Pinta (*T. carateum*) is a disease endemic in Central and South America.

CLINICAL FEATURES

In *yaws* the initial lesion (yaw) is commoner on the lower limbs; it is papillomatous in form and painless. A painful lesion may occur on the sole of the foot (crab yaw). Within three to six

* *e.g.* Yaws and syphilis treponemes differ in their effects when inoculated into hamsters.

weeks of its appearance a generalised eruption occurs. The various types of lesion are similar to those seen in syphilis: macules, squames, maculopapular, nodular, plaques and papillomata; lesions are also noted on the palms and soles and on the mucosae. The bones are not infrequently affected, chiefly the periosteum,

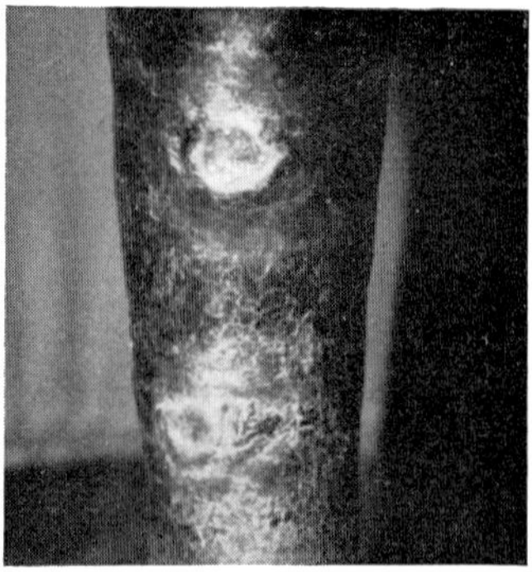

FIG. 156.

Active lesions of late Yaws on the lower leg.

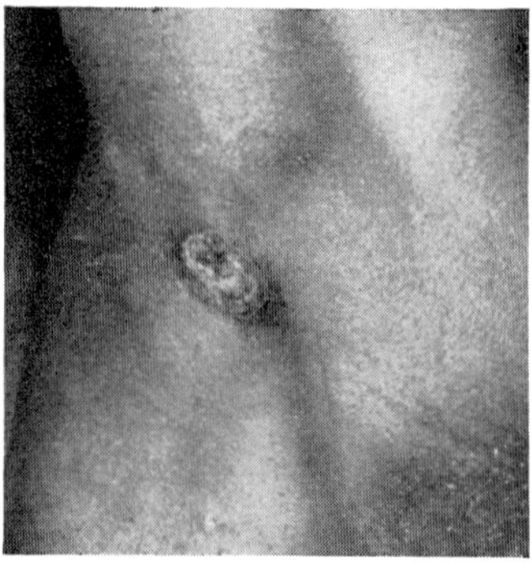

FIG. 157.

Typical thin scar of healed Yaws on the hip.

and in particular the long bones. An hypertrophic osteo-periostitis affects the nasal maxilla, giving rise to a characteristic appearance. In the late stages, cutaneous lesions tend to be plaque-like, nodular or ulcerative, and extensive disfigurement may arise from lesions involving deeper tissues or bone.

Bejel. The lesions of generalised type are not dissimilar from those of syphilis, and may be accompanied by laryngitis and osteocopic pains. Late lesions may involve subcutaneous tissue and bone and result in destruction of deep tissue with disfigurement.

Pinta. The initial lesions occurs on the lower limbs, followed later by a generalised eruption, similar to but on the whole drier in type than the other syphilides or yaws. The disease is chronic and mild.

Treatment

The non-syphilitic treponematoses respond well to parenteral penicillin. The treatment is usually by a long-acting penicillin such as benethamine, or procaine penicillin given by intramuscular injection, at suitable intervals, to a total of six million units.

SELECTED BIBLIOGRAPHY FOR NON-VENEREAL DISORDERS OF THE GENITALIA

HERPES SIMPLEX (GENITALIS)

Hutfield, D. C., Wasley, G. D. & Gray, E. (1967). *Br. J. vener. Dis.* **43,** 48.

Parker, J. D. & Banatvala, J. E. (1967). *Br. J. vener. Dis.* **43,** 212.

Virus Papilloma (condylomata acuminata)

See Teokharov, B. E. (Selected bibliography for Ch. 8).

Aphthosis

Masterton, G. (1965). *Br. J. vener. Dis.* **41,** 292.

Lehner, T. (1967). *Br. med. J.* **1,** 465.

Non-syphilitic Treponematoses

YAWS

World Health Organization Bulletin, (1967). No. 36.

BEJEL

Hudson, E. H. (1957). Edinburgh: Livingstone.

CHAPTER 11

Psychiatric Aspects of Venereal Disease

Fear of venereal disease may bring a patient to their doctor and a proportion of such patients will have a psychiatric illness provoked by this fear or anxiety. The way in which fear of a venereal disease presents makes many of these cases of psychiatric illness look alike: thus the diagnosis is seldom obvious. A wide variety of psychiatric disorders may present in this fashion, and although true 'phobia' is not rare, the term venerophobia should be used only when the characteristics of an obsession are present.

AETIOLOGY

Feelings of fear or guilt play a large part in the evolution of these disorders; together with other factors, such as the constitutional endowment and the general physical health of the patient.

The conditions likely to be met with most frequently are the anxiety syndromes and the depressive illnesses. The commonest presenting symptoms are anxiety, obsession, genital pain and itching without organic cause, depression, impotence and frigidity. The less common symptoms include delusions, auditory hallucinations, panic attacks, suicidal ideas, phantom genital swelling or diminution in size. Other categories of patient may include the obsessional, hysterical, psychopathic personality, the schizophrenic patient or one with organic cerebral disorder.

Anxiety is to be regarded as abnormal when it is provoked by an inadequate cause or when it is abnormally persistent and accompanied by physical symptoms. It may disguise a depressive state: depression becomes a psychiatric symptom when there is an affect of sadness and gloom without adequate cause. The depressive illness is usually distinguished as reactive, endogenous or involutional in type. Suicidal ideas are commonest in the depressive illnesses. True phobia may appear in a variety of disorders; most commonly in endogenous depression, but also in anxiety neurosis, obsessional states, or hysteria. A schizophrenic reaction may be accompanied by delusions, hallucinations or paranoid features: for example, a patient believes that his syphilis, non-existent in fact, has become a general topic of conversation with those about him.

TREATMENT

Many of these patients with psychiatric illness are mild cases, and a high proportion are susceptible of improvement either spontaneously or with the help of drug treatment and supportive psychotherapy. In particular the prognosis is good in patients with anxiety syndromes or depression, most of whom can receive treatment in the clinic, or from their own doctor if he has the time to give to them. Severe cases and those with psychoses or obsessional traits require to be treated by a psychiatrist.

SELECTED BIBLIOGRAPHY FOR PSYCHIATRIC ASPECTS

Kite, E. & Grimble, A. (1963). *Br. J. vener. Dis.* **39,** 173.

Siboulet, A. (1960). *Br. J. vener. Dis.* **36,** 118.

See also under 'Psychology of sexually promiscuous patients' in selected bibliography for Chapter 12 (Epidemiology).—Palmer, M. (1949).

CHAPTER 12

Epidemiology of Venereal Diseases

Epidemiology is the science and study of infectious disease; its prevalence, variation, recurrence, and factors responsible for its transmission and control. In this study we look also for information about the behaviour of persons 'at risk'. Many of these disorders are due to known infective agents; some of them, for example gonorrhoea, require the existence of sexual promiscuity in order to spread the infection in the community. Others may arise *de novo* in the genito-urinary tract, subsequently to be transmitted sexually, but not necessarily through 'promiscuous' sexual activity. In the above context, we are particularly concerned with those diseases which carry the greatest dangers to health: the chronic disease of syphilis; and acute gonorrhoea with its greater danger, at present, for women than men.

INCIDENCE

The incidence of these diseases over the years has been a fluctuating one (exemplified by gonorrhoea for England and Wales (Fig. 158); and the present increase in infection is not confined to any country or to any particular part of the world. It is due to a great many factors: sociological, psychological (behavioural) and biological; the conduct of human beings in the community, and certain characteristics of the infecting organisms themselves, are the most important of these. Social factors, which most affect trends, are chiefly wars, population movements and economic instability or depression. Personal and psychological factors are many; and they tend to arise out of the formation of irresponsible attitudes through the presence of an unfavourable and adverse environment in childhood.

CONTROL

There are three ways of controlling an infectious disease: to treat where possible every acutely infected person or chronic

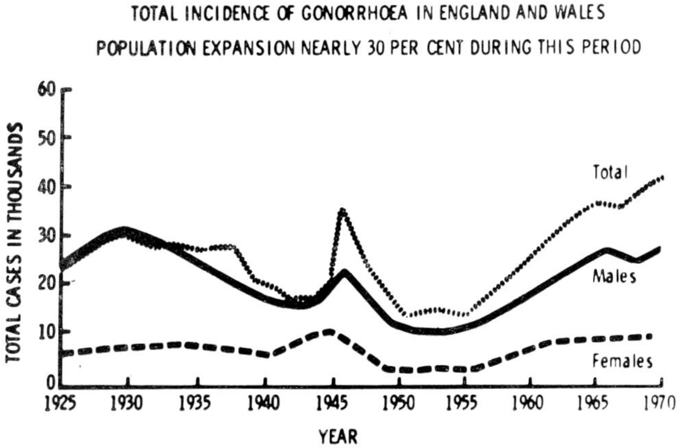

FIG. 158.

Incidence of sexually infected conditions shown to have a rhythmic pattern as reflected by that for acute gonorrhoea—male: female ratio about 4:1.

carrier; to control closely the route or manner by which the disease is transmitted; and then to induce an immunity in the population at risk, preferably an active artificial immunity. None of these tasks is easy when we are confronted with a sexually transmitted illness. The last of the three methods enumerated is the best but is extremely difficult in this context, difficult because not many members of a community would concede that they were 'bad risks' and seek immunisation on this account. There is doubt too whether an effective 'vaccine' can be prepared against the larger type of micro-organism with which we are dealing. The sole means, therefore, of keeping control over these diseases is by attempting to find and treat all infected persons, and by ensuring that the organisms are susceptible to the drugs used against the disease.

In order to obtain the co-operation of the patient all services should be given free. Clinics for the diagnosis and treatment of venereal diseases should be strategically placed in hospital outpatient departments, 'confidential' in the way they are conducted and handle their documents. However, undue secrecy achieves nothing.

A small number of patients with a serious disorder such as syphilis will neither attend a clinic nor visit a doctor privately. In these circumstances Public Health departments should use their trained staff to find and persuade them to attend for treatment. This is urgent when such patients are, for example, in contact with children or, less importantly, food-handling, or if they are expectant mothers.

It is illegal at the present time to advertise medicines for the treatment of venereal disease; and it is noteworthy that campaigns launched to bring these diseases before the public notice have tended to breed anxiety amongst a portion of that public. Penal measures to prevent the spread of infection, or legal compulsion for the attendance of an infected person at a clinic, have not brought success: we may compare France, Russia and Holland in this respect, the former two countries possessing legal compulsion, the last not, neither being the better off. The sources of infection, where there are means for compulsion to attend a clinic, become even harder to discover and even less co-operative when they are found and persuaded to receive treatment. The war-time Emergency Regulation (33b 1942) was one move this country made towards compulsion: it was rarely if ever used, and lapsed after the Second World War.

PROSTITUTION

Prostitutes are only one group amongst those acting as carriers of venereal infection. Flexner thought that the incidence of infectious syphilis in Viennese prostitutes at the beginning of this century was 50 per cent. In recent years, with syphilis much less common, Keighley showed that the incidence of gonorrhoea in prostitutes entering Holloway gaol, up to the age of 20 years, was 40 per cent. Venereal infection is contracted from a prostitute by less than 20 per cent of men with gonorrhoea in this country. Although the figures from many European countries are similar, those from Asian countries are much higher. The proportion of men who visit prostitutes rises with age. The event of marriage appears to make no decisive difference to the sexual behaviour pattern of many males whose sexual activities have included regular liaisons with prostitutes. Many of these men come from broken homes and appear to be less able to sustain lasting emotional relationships, seeking speedy fulfilment of their desires and transient satisfaction in this manner.

SEXUAL BEHAVIOUR PATTERNS

In this country 80 per cent of men contracting gonorrhoea do so through liaisons with comparative strangers, but only 25 per cent of women behave like this: 40 per cent of the men with gonorrhoea are itinerant, the women very seldom so: most of the men admit to drinking alcohol before coitus; of the women only one in four do, according to one survey.

This illustrates what is generally known concerning the different pattern of sexual activity of the two sexes. Anthropology, and, more recently, the work of Kinsey and his colleagues, have clarified this subject for us. In the individual male, the ability to indulge in frequent or continuous sexual activity is closely related to physiological potency, which is highest in the late 'teens and tends to fall after the age of 35; but there is a very wide variation in potency between individuals. Thus the physiological drive towards some sexual outlet is very great indeed in certain males, especially in those below the age of 25, to many of whom the sex act assumes little or no emotional importance. The largest age-group of men attending the clinic is that in the early to middle twenties.

The pattern of sexual outlet in most women is almost entirely different: whereas the potential amount of sexual activity in the majority of men is maximal in their early twenties, it tends to build up slowly in most women, many of whom may not arrive at any regular sexual activity until the late twenties or beyond. Their sexual capacity, starting slowly, does not appear greatly to diminish over the years.

For these and other psycho-social reasons, a given number of young men will perforce always consort with a smaller number of young women, who, if they are carriers of infection, will be in a position to spread it widely.

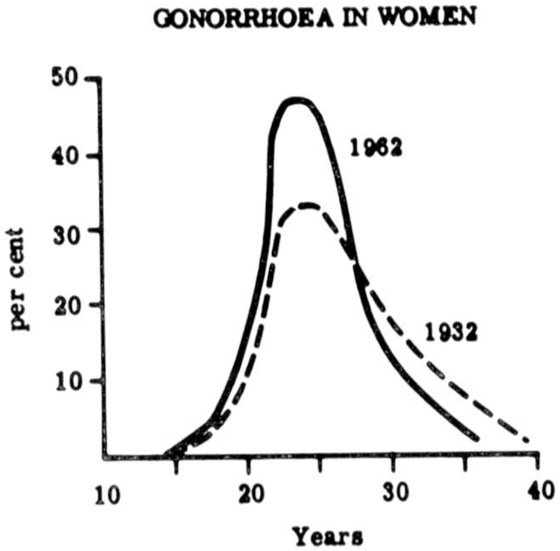

FIG. 159.
Contrasts incidence in women for 1932 and 1962.

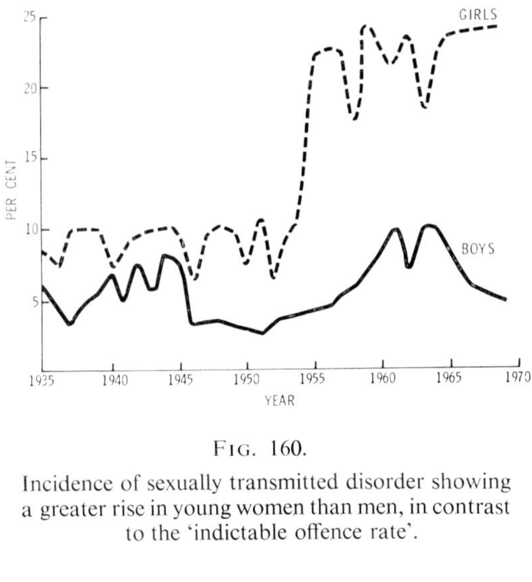

FIG. 160.
Incidence of sexually transmitted disorder showing a greater rise in young women than men, in contrast to the 'indictable offence rate'.

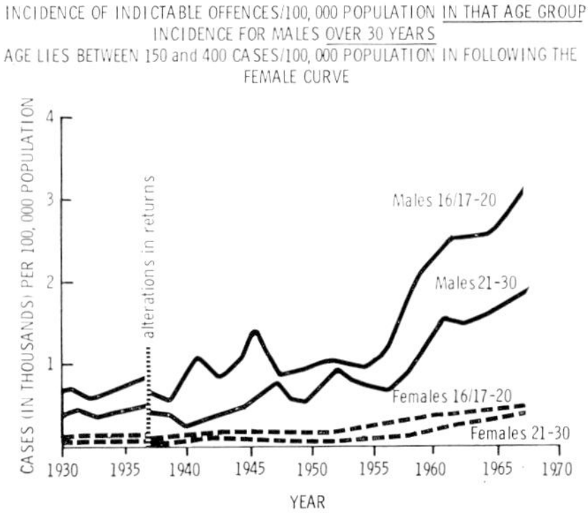

FIG. 161.

Indictable Offence Rate, demonstrating that the 'rise' is a phenomenon mainly confined to young males.

Distinction must be made between the circumspect, premarital relationship and the promiscuous one, promiscuity in this context being defined as a casual sexual liason without emotional attachment. The individuals persistently indulging in promiscuous relations have faulty environmental and home backgrounds rather than any personality defects. Habitual promiscuity may be looked upon as a form of delinquent behaviour, and this would appear to be true of the hard core of young people who practise it to satisfy their need for emotional recognition. This may be seen especially in young girls, who indulge in it much as the boys indulge in 'gang' pursuits and petty crime. Promiscuity, delinquency and crime are not infrequently found together. But it is noteworthy that promiscuity and delinquency both diminish with age (Figs. 159–161).

Other aspects of promiscuity in sexual relations include male homosexuality, seafarers, and migrants, itinerants or travellers in general. This problem is unlikely to diminish as the world's population increases, and there is now greater individual and group movements across the globe for either work or pleasure or both.

The various social aspects of the transmission of these venereal infections which depend on a promiscuous sexual activity, studied together with the problems of control, give little cause for complacency. Education on the nature of these diseases, about the existence of the chronic disease of syphilis and of the dangers of gonorrhoea in women, should be obligatory in all young people, though in manner sensitive and tactful, along with sex education. None of these disorders is untreatable, and none should bear a stigma.

SELECTED BIBLIOGRAPHY FOR EPIDEMIOLOGY

FAILURE TO CONTROL

Rees, E. (1964). *Br. med. J.* **1,** 47.
Willcox, R. R. (1967) *Acta dermato-vener., Stockh.* **47,** 65.
Juhlint Liden S. (1968). *Wld Hlth Org. V.D. trans.* No. 352.

PSYCHOLOGY OF SEXUALLY PROMISCUOUS PATIENTS

Keighley, E. (1963). *Br. J. vener. Dis.* **39,** 278.
O'Hare, J. (1960). *Br. J. vener. Dis.* **36,** 122.
Gibbens, T. & Siberman, M. (1960). *Br. J. vener. Dis.* **36,** 113.
Knobel, M. (1962). *U.S. Dept. Publ. Hlth Rep.*, p. 407.
Whittkower, E. (1948). *Br. J. vener. Dis.* **24,** 59.
Palmer, M. (1949). *Br. J. vener. Dis.* **25,** 124.

VENEREAL DISEASE IN PROSTITUTES

Gibbens, T. (1957). *Br. J. Delinq.* **8,** 3.
Rosenthal, T. & Kershner, G. (1948). *Am. J. Syph. Neurol.* **32,** 256.
Raymondis, L. (1963). *Rev. int. Crimin.* **17,** 87.
Laird, S. (1956). *Br. J. vener. Dis.* **32,** 181.

HOMOSEXUALITY IN VENEREAL DISEASE

Jefferies, J. (1956). *Br. J. vener. Dis.* **32,** 17.
Hermans, E. H. & Cock, P. de (1963). *Dermatologica, Basel,* **127,** 278.
Ketterer, W. (1964). *J. Am. med. Ass.* **188,** 811.

SEAFARERS AND VENEREAL DISEASE

Idsoe, O. & Guthe, T. (1963). *Bull Wld Hlth Org.* **29,** 773.
Magussen, B. & Otterland, A. (1964). *Acta dermato-venereol., Stockh.* **44,** 141.

MIGRATION AND VENEREAL DISEASE
Brown, W. (1950). *Br. J. vener. Dis.* **36,** 49.
Willcox, R. (1964). *Wld Hlth Org. trans.* No. 323.

LEGISLATION IN EUROPE CONCERNED WITH VENEREAL DISEASE
De moerloose, J. & Rahm, H. (1964). *Acta dermato-venereol. Stockh.* **44,** 146.

SEXUAL BEHAVIOUR: ANTHROPOLOGICAL
Ford, C., Beach, F. & Crew, F. (1952). Eyre, Spottiswoode, London.
Matinowski, B. (1926). Routledge, London, 1927.

SEXUAL BEHAVIOUR: CONTEMPORARY
Various authors (1961). Education, London.
Quaker View (1964). Friends' House.
Kinsey, A. *et al.* (1958). Saunders, London & N.Y.
Schofield, M. (1965). Longmans, London.

Part 4

Special Techniques

CHAPTER 13

Clinical and Laboratory Procedures

INTRODUCTION

A knowledge of procedures such as venepuncture, lumbar puncture, urethrescopy and prostatic massage is required for routine work in a venereal disease clinic. Urethral irrigation, and irrigation of the bladder, are hardly ever carried out today.

It is as well, also, to have some experience of the serological test procedures used for the detection of specific antibodies, and it is essential to understand the staining and cultural methods commonly employed for the isolation of micro-organisms. Oil immersion microscopy, with a light source and a $\frac{1}{12}$ objective lens, is used for scanning the stained smears; a dark-ground condenser is inserted in place of the ordinary one when a 'live' field is being scanned, for example for *Trichomonas vaginalis* or *Treponema pallidum*.

CLINICAL PROCEDURES

BLOOD-TAKING

Venepuncture. Collection of blood in adults is most conveniently obtained from a prominent vessel, the usual site being the antecubital fossa. The arm should be fully extended, palm upwards. The skin is exposed from the wrist to near the shoulder. A rubber tourniquet is applied to the upper arm, and adjusted tightly to constrict the veins. The patient then clenches the hand: if the veins do not become prominent the patient unclenches and clenches the hand slowly, whilst the arm is massaged firmly from the wrist upwards.

A suitable vein having been selected and the overlying skin sterilised with spirit or antiseptic such as 1 per cent hibitane, the vein is fixed by the thumb of the left hand, which is placed an inch or so distal to the proposed site of puncture, and the skin drawn taut. The point of a stout hypodermic needle attached to a 5 ml. or 10 ml. syringe is pushed rapidly bevel upwards through the skin, in the mid-line of the vein, and is made to travel through the subcutaneous tissue along the line of the vein, picking up and entering it. The syringe is then fixed with the left hand and the patient's blood withdrawn. The tourniquet is released, the needle removed, and the patient instructed to press firmly for a minute or two on a small pad of cotton wool placed over the site of the puncture, in order to prevent haematoma.

In very young children, blood may be obtained from a scalp vein or the anterior jugular vein, constriction of the vein proximally being obtained by pressure from the finger of an assistant. Alternatively, blood may be obtained by '*heel-stab*'. Pressure is applied immediately below the knee. The skin over the pad of the heel is thoroughly cleansed, sterilised with spirit or suitable antiseptic and allowed to dry. Incision is made into the pad of the heel with a smart stab of a sharp-pointed tenotome, care being taken to avoid bone. The ooze of blood is facilitated by firmly stroking the leg downwards from the knee.

A minimum of 2 ml. of blood should be collected in a small bottle or a Wright's capsule.

LUMBAR PUNCTURE

The needle is introduced between the third and fourth, or fourth and fifth, spinous processes of the lumbar vertebrae, and the specimen of cerebrospinal fluid is obtained after entering the subarachnoid space. No special equipment is needed apart from a lumbar puncture needle of, for example, the Harris or the Dattner pattern. The latter has a fine inner needle occluded by a stilette; but the Harris needle is suitably fine, and post-operative headache is more likely to be due to factors in the patient or operator than to this needle.

Preparation of the Patient

No special preparation of the patient, other than cleansing the skin, is necessary. In the case of a nervous patient, premedication with a barbiturate (phenobarbitone 30–60 mg.) or pethidine

(10–30 mg.) may be advisable. Lumbar puncture is carried out with the patient sitting up or lying on the side, according to the individual preference of the operator. The skin over the lumbar spines is washed with 1·0 per cent hibitane or soap and water, dried and sterilised with tincture of iodine. It is of assistance to delineate the iliac crests with this antiseptic. The subsequent stages in the operation are: (1) Bend the patient forward, flexing the head, thereby separating as widely as possible the spinous processes of the lumbar vertebrae. (2) The tip of the spinous process of the fourth lumbar vertebra lies in the horizontal plane joining the highest points of the iliac crests: this point is determined. (3) The interspace between the third and fourth, or fourth and fifth, lumbar spines is infiltrated with 1 per cent novocain. An intracutaneous wheal is first made in the mid-line of the body, and the needle then directed deeply through the ligaments towards the meninges, infiltrating the tissues with anaesthetic. Two to three ml. may be required. (4) The spinal puncture needle, which has been sterilised, is then directed horizontally through the skin and interspinous ligament towards the theca. The needle is gradually inserted until a sudden loss of resistance indicates that the point has penetrated the theca. In the event of the needle striking the bone it should be partially withdrawn and reinserted at a slightly different angle according to the position of the lumbar spines. The stilette is now withdrawn and the first few drops of spinal fluid allowed to escape. From 4 to 6 ml. of the fluid should be collected in a sterile test-tube for examination. Very slow, or intermittent flow may indicate that the needle point has not completely entered the theca, or that the eye is obstructed by one of the filaments of the cauda equina. This may be remedied by partial rotation of the needle, or by inserting it slightly further.

During puncture the pressure of the cerebrospinal fluid varies normally from 60 to 150 mm. with the patient on the side. In syphilitic paresis (general paralysis of the insane) and in many cases of meningeal reaction the pressure may be markedly increased. Nervousness of the patient, compression over the jugular veins, or interference with free respiration also result in increase of pressure. A free rise and fall with compression of the jugular veins indicates an unobstructed flow of the cerebrospinal fluid.

After collection of the specimen the patient should rest in the prone position with the pelvis raised on a pillow for the rest of that day. These measures decrease the post-operative leakage of the cerebrospinal fluid which is the cause of post-puncture headache. The headache can be mild or extremely severe, and is frequently associated with nausea and vomiting. It may last for only a few hours or persist for seven to ten days. Established 'headache' disappears when the patient lies down with the head low, but recurs on rising. In milder cases relief may follow the administration of aspirin, phenacetin and caffeine tablets, or salicylate alone in doses of 0·65 g. four-hourly. In severe cases pethidine (10 mg.) is required for relief.

After collection of the specimen the following observations are made:—(1) Colour and appearance of the fluid. (2) Cell count. (3) Increase of total protein and globulin. (4) The Wassermann reaction. (5) The gold-sol (Lange) or similar reaction (p. 81).

Normal cerebrospinal fluid is clear and colourless and has a specific gravity of 1,004 to 1,008. The number of cells varies from 0 to 5 per c.mm. These cells consist of large and small lymphocytes, with occasionally a large mononuclear cell. A lymphocyte count between 5 and 10 per c.mm. is considered suspicious; more than 10 is definitely pathological if the specimen has not been contaminated by blood during the puncture. Normally globulin is absent or only the faintest trace can be demonstrated.

PROSTATIC MASSAGE AND COLLECTION OF SECRETION

See p. 142.

INTRAMUSCULAR INJECTION

All patients should be asked whether they have received the drug before, if they suffered any ill-effects from it in the past, and whether they have suffered from an allergy. The site generally chosen for intramuscular injection is the upper and outer, gluteal quadrant.

The patient preferably stands erect. It is important to secure relaxation of the muscles at the site into which injection is to be made. The patient should have the knee bent slightly, relaxing the gluteal muscles on the injected side. The skin over the site is cleaned with spirit or 1 per cent hibitane. A stout intramuscular needle is held by its mount between the forefinger and thumb, the tip of the middle finger resting on the shaft close to the mount, and it is stabbed smartly into the chosen site. Care should be taken that the iliac bone is not struck. The introduction of the needle should be painless. It is important to wait for a few moments to make certain that the point has not punctured a blood vessel (if this has occurred partial withdrawal and re-insertion is necessary); the syringe is then attached and the drug injected. Deep rotary massage of the area of injection should now be madc to distribute the drug through the tissues; this also lessens subsequent pain or tenderness. Successive injections should be given on alternate sides and the site should be varied slightly on each occasion.

URETHROSCOPY

In the investigation of persistent infections of the male urethra, visual inspection of the urethra and its glandular openings affords information which cannot otherwise be gained. The urethroscope is also of value in the investigation of endocervicitis complicating vulvo-vaginitis in young girls, in the tests of cure of gonorrhoea in the adult, and, to a lesser extent, for intra-urethral operative procedures in the male or female.

The urethroscope has an obturator to facilitate introduction, lighting and magnifying visual systems, which are usually combined, and an attachment to permit distension of the urethra by air or water pressure. The lighting system may be external or internal: either from a tube, when the visual field is illuminated by a pencil of light reflected by a mirror or prism; or from a miniature electric bulb, mounted on a slender stem positioned within the instrument near the internal opening of the tube as in the Harrison's urethroscope commonly used today in this country.

Special water-distension urethroscopes (such as the Geringer) may be preferable for a view of the structures in the membranous or prostatic urethra. Urethroscopy is practically painless, and in anterior urethroscopy the use of local anaesthesia should where possible be avoided because of the alteration caused in the appearance of the mucous membrane: in posterior urethroscopy, despite the mucosal anaemia caused, local analgesia is essential owing to the risk of syncope in the patient.

Urethroscopy enables the inspection of the epithelium of the male urethra when viral urethritis is suspected (p. 141), or where urethritis fails to resolve in either sex; in the diagnosis of local complications in the male such as littritis, posterior urethritis accompanying prostatitis; and also where there is suspected stricture.

Urethroscopy is inadvisable in the presence of acute inflammation, owing to pain, the risk of spreading the infection locally, or of forcing bacteria into the circulation from trauma to a blood vessel.

Technique of Anterior Urethroscopy

The patient should not have micturated for three hours. The rules of antisepsis and asepsis should be observed. The male patient may lie flat on an examination couch with the pelvis slightly raised on a firm, flat cushion; the female is placed in the lithotomy position.

The urethroscopic tube, with its obturator in position, is lubricated and introduced into the urethra, the tip being directed towards and reaching the junction of the bulbous and membranous urethrae. The obturator is withdrawn. If any free bleeding caused by the introduction of the cannula is not immediately controlled by gentle pressure, it is wise to withdraw the cannula and defer examination to a later date owing to the possible risk of embolism and introduction of bacteria when using air pressure. The lighting and visual systems are attached to the cannula, and, as the instrument is slowly withdrawn, each successive field from the bulb to the external meatus is carefully studied.

On looking down a urethroscope, when no air dilatation has been applied, the walls of the male urethra are in apposition, the mucous membrane being thrown into longitudinal folds, giving a 'wheel-spoke' appearance to the radiation of the folds of the urethra from the central lumen.

The application of air pressure causes ballooning of the urethra. Besides enabling one to assess its resiliency, this widens the field of view and stretches the openings of the Littré's gland ducts and lacunae of Morgagni, making these structures more prominent.

Urethroscopic Appearance in the Male

The mucous membrane of the healthy urethra shows considerable variation in colour, not only in different individuals, but also in different portions of the same urethra. The colour progressively deepens proximally, from yellowish-pink in the region of the glans penis to a full red transfused with slight yellow in the bulb. The colour is dependent upon the richness of the blood supply to the vessels which, running longitudinally in the submucous tissues, impart to the mucosa its characteristic hue and vascular striations. The smooth epithelial surface of the urethra lubricated by the alkaline secretion of the Littré's glands has a characteristic lustre.

In the *bulbous urethra* the central collapsed lumen appears as a transverse slit; the longitudinal folds of the urethra and the vascular striations are well marked. Lucanae of Morgagni are recognised as small V-shaped pouches with a broad end directed towards the meatus. Littré's glands are numerous, though often invisible in health.

The orifice of the membranous urethra and the openings of Cowper's ducts can be well seen in the distended urethra. The former appears as a horizontal crescentic hooded slit. The ducts of Cowper's glands open on the floor of the bulbous urethra, and appear as two pear-shaped orifices lying usually on either side of the mid-line.

In the *penile urethra* the collapsed lumen is small and circular, the mucous surface of rose-pink colour, the longitudinal folds of the mucous membrane and the vascular striations forming a regular stellate pattern. There is marked elasticity of the urethral, and air distension shows up the submucosal circular muscular rings. The lacunae of Morgagni are seen in the roof in the mid-line, and on either side lies a chain of Littré's glands.

In the region of the *fossa navicularis* the lumen forms a small, vertical ovoid slit, the mucous membrane is of pale yellow colour and shows no longitudinal folds or vascular striations. This area is almost inelastic. The lacuna magna is visible on the roof about one inch proximal to the external urinary meatus.

Urethroscopic Appearances in the Diseased Male Urethra

The anterior urethroscopic picture in acute urethritis shows alterations in the colour, lustre and appearance of the mucous membrane, alterations in the elasticity of the urethra, and changes affecting the lacunae of Morgagni and the glands of Littré.

According to the existing degree of fibrosis which occurs, infiltrations may be noted. In a soft infiltration, the mucous membrane is at first red, often with darker erosions of the epithelium which bleed easily. At this stage the elasticity of the urethra, in response to air insufflation, is unaltered. Littré's glands are usually involved.

Further organisation of fibrous tissue in the affected area leads to less congestion of the epithelium, sluggish dilatation under air pressure, and the appearance of fibrous streaks in the mucosa.

Later the mucous membrane becomes blanched, the columnar epithelium is replaced by the squamous type, the surface is uneven, and often there is a patchy loss of epithelium. The urethra becomes highly inelastic from the alteration of the sub-mucosal tissue (stage of hard infiltration).

Involvement of the *glands* of Litré and the lacunae of Morgagni is an invariable accompaniment of urethritis. Littré's glands secrete a clear mucus; infection is indicated by the exudate altering to muco-pus. The openings of the gland ducts, normally inconspicuous, show as angry red points, often raised and surrounded by areas of hyperaemia. Occlusion of the ducts may result in abscess formation or cysts. Deposits of fibrous tissue are often observed surrounding the orifices of the gland ducts. Similar pathological changes are observed in the lacunae of Morgagni.

Resolution of soft infiltrations and of the glandular involvement may follow therapy. This does not occur with the fibrous type.

Inflammatory changes of the *prostatic urethra* cause a peculiar dull, velvety, cyanotic colour of the mucosa, most marked over the verumontanum; the prostatic utricle is gaping and discharges muco-pus or pus. The orifices of the common ejaculatory ducts and prostatic ducts become slightly raised and hyperaemic. In the latter stages of infection, sub-epithelial fibrosis occurs, causing irregular sclerotic plaques or granulating areas on the mucous membrane. The verumontanum becomes shrunken and flattened, and the orifices of the ejaculatory ducts shrink and become stenosed.

Urethroscopy in the Female

With the patient in the Trendelenburg position the cannula, with its obturator fitted, is passed along the urethra until the tip enters the bladder. The obturator is withdrawn, and the bladder emptied by a soft rubber catheter passed through the endoscopic tube. The visual and lighting systems are now attached and the trigone of the bladder inspected. As the urethroscope is gradually withdrawn, the vesical sphincter can be observed to close behind it. The mucous membrane of the healthy urethra is smooth, lustrous, of a pale pink colour, and is thrown into longitudinal folds. Glandular openings are not often visible. Immediately proximal to the external meatus one sees the orifices of Skene's tubules on the floor and sides of the urethra.

The pathological conditions found in gonococcal infection of the female urethra are closely similar to those of the male, namely, injection and oedema of the mucous membrane, submucous infiltrations, and infection of the glandular structures.

URINARY INSPECTION

As a clinical guide to inflammatory disorder of the lower genito-urinary tract, inspection of the urine in clean cylindrical glasses is of the greatest assistance.

It yields more information in men than in women, in whom the shortness of the urethra and a variable amount of contamination from the vulva to some extent limits its usefulness. Furthermore, urethritis in women, unless acute or unless part of a post-menopausal condition, is frequently accompanied by cystitis.

In men the early stages of urethral infection present with increased epithelial exfoliation, rapidly followed in acute infections by the appearance of leucocytes. Early signs in the first glass or urine are of small desquamated *flakes*, round or comma-shaped, consisting of epithelial cells and leucocytes. The formation of much pus accompanied by a *haze* in the first glass of urine indicates inflammation which is limited to the anterior two-thirds of the urethra. When there is severe inflammation chunks of débris may be seen in the urine; these are always heavy and sink to the bottom of the glass.

Infection, which comes to involve the ducts and glands of Littré, Cowper's gland, vesicles or the prostate, results in small *threads* in the urine, consisting of leucocytes, epithelial cells, débris and mucus. Long threads are evidence of infection of the prostate gland and ducts and the vesicles.

A two-glass urinary haze with or without débris indicates posterior urethral inflammation in men, or bladder infection in men and women. A light haze in both glasses also accompanies a heavy bacteruria, and phosphaturia.

PASSAGE OF SOUNDS

Sounds are of two types, straight and curved. They should be sterilised by boiling for 15 minutes, or cleaned with 1 per cent Hibitane before use, and lubricated just before insertion with jelly or soft paraffin.

The technique for insertion of the straight metal sound offers no difficulty. Its principal use lies in the detection of littritis and in the dilatation of anterior strictures.

The curved metal sound should be inserted so that the curved tip lies in line with the long axis of the urethra the whole way. In order to do this the handle and shaft of the sound are held nearly at right-angles to the long axis of the urethra, and the insertions made until the tip of the sound approaches the posterior urethra and pubic ligament; at this point the handle is swung round and near vertically in order that the curve of the sound may lie upwards, its concavity towards the pubis, at which point the sound will travel without difficulty along the posterior urethra and into the bladder.

LABORATORY PROCEDURES

Staining Methods

Gram's Stain

Place a thin smear of material on a glass slide; heat in a flame briefly in order to 'fix' the material. Stain with 2 per cent crystal violet for half a minute or less; then add Gram's iodine (to fix violet stain) for the same duration. Wash off with tap-water. Decolourise with acetone-alcohol mixture (proportion unimportant) until colour ceases to run off. Wash in tap-water. One half of the bacterial kingdom retains the violet stain after washing with acetone and alcohol, the other does not. The former is a 'Gram positive' organism, the latter 'Gram negative'.

Counterstain with acid-dye, *e.g.* 2 per cent carbol fuchsin or neutral red, for 60 seconds. Wash in tap-water. Blot and dry.

Suitable for all bacterial work.

Giemsa Stain

This consists of differing mixtures of methylene blue and eosin (Azur).

Fix smears in methanol three minutes. Stain with 1 part stain and 10 parts buffer (pH 7·0) for one hour. Wash with buffer and differentiate 30 seconds. Blot and dry in air.

Another method may be used, warming the slide before staining for 15 minutes.

Suitable for inclusion bodies, and many parasites.

Loeffler's Alkaline Methylene Blue (used when polychromatic with age).

Stain for 45 minutes or longer. Wash in tap-water. May be used over a Gram's stain.

Suitable for *Trichomonas vaginalis.*

FLUORESCENT TECHNIQUES

These techniques are used to attach chemically fluorescent dyes either to antibodies or to micro-organisms, which can then be identified when examined microscopically under ultraviolet light. The technique is chiefly used in venereology to identify *treponemal antibody* in the FTA test, and *gonococci* in smears of exudate and secretion.

When using the direct staining technique (which is simpler but less sensitive than the indirect) for identification of *N. gonorrhoeae*, the smear of secretion is first dried in the air and fixed by heating. The anti-gonococcal serum conjugate (with rhodamine dye or fluorescein) is diluted with buffer, mixed and placed in minimal amounts upon the slide, which is incubated in a moist chamber at 37° C. for three-quarters of an hour. The slide is then washed in buffer for 10 minutes, blotted and dried in the air, and subsequently examined by dark-ground illumination, under oil immersion, using an ultra-violet light source.

Cultural Methods

Fermentation and oxidase reactions, to determine whether or not a *Neisseria gonorrhoeae* is present. The medium consists of peptone 20 g., sodium chloride 5 g., distilled water 900 ml.; make pink to phenolphthalein and adjust to pH 7·6, and add 100 ml. digest broth. Add 2·5 per cent agar powder and sterilise.

For use, melt 100 ml. of medium and add 5 ml. sterile guinea-pig serum and 10 ml. 10 per cent refined sugar. Make up in sterile slopes. Fermentation by the bacterium results in acidity with a colour change from pink to yellow.

N. gonorrhoeae ferments glucose but not maltose.

Oxidase reaction for Neisseria: add a loopful of fresh 1 per cent aqueous tetra-methyl-p-phenylenediamine hydrochloride to colonies on blood agar plate. A positive reaction occurs if the colony rapidly develops a purple colour; several Neisseria give this result.

STUART'S TRANSPORT MEDIUM

This is a useful non-nutrient material for a swab carrying bacteria or trichomonas. It consists of buffered semi-solid agar, and contains sodium thioglycollate and methylene blue, in order to maintain an anaerobic environment. The swabs should be impregnated with charcoal.

Serological Techniques

SEROLOGICAL TESTING FOR SYPHILITIC ANTIBODIES

Whole dried blood 5–15 ml. are allowed to clot. The specimen may be centrifuged before the serum is drawn off with a pipette for use, and then decomplemented (inactivated) by heating at 56° C. for half an hour.

The most widely performed technique for detecting serum antibodies in venereal disorders is that of *complement fixation*. It is used in syphilis for two of the tests, the *Wassermann reaction* (W.R.) and the *Reiter protein complement fixation test* (RPCFT); in gonorrhoea for the *gonococcal complement fixation test* (GCFT); and for the detection of *virus antibodies* in such disorders as lymphogranuloma venereum.

Notes as a guide to the technique of the *Wassermann reaction*:—

Complement fixing system: one-fifth of a volume inactivated serum; one volume antigen (cholestinised alcoholic extract of ox heart muscle), one volume guinea-pig complement (1·5 minimal haemolytic doses) and one volume normal saline are incubated at 37° C. for one hour, together with a 'control tube' containing one-fifth of a volume serum, one volume complement and 2 volumes saline.

Haemolytic system for detecting unfixed (free) complement: one volume of 2·5 per cent suspension of sheep red cells plus five minimal doses of amboceptor (immune body in rabbit anti-serum to sheep red cells, obtained by repeatedly injecting rabbit with sheep cells) are added to each tube, and the tubes then incubated for a further half-hour.

When examined for haemolysis: *no* haemolysis indicates that there is *no* free complement equal positive W.R. Presence of haemolysis equals negative W.R.

The *Kahn flocculation*, like *Price's precipitation*, reaction does not make use of complement fixation. The Kahn, or Price's, test is used as a second standard test for syphilis. These two tests are commonly performed in a quantitative manner thus giving a measure of the titre (or degree of positivity) of the serum.

Three tubes are used containing two volumes antigen and one volume inactivated serum (one volume equals 0·15 ml.). The tubes are well shaken (in the Kahn test for five minutes), and 10 volumes normal saline is then added to each tube, which is again shaken. Flocculation is noted by examining the tube on the slant and finding floccules (discrete particles seen with a hand lens). The titre is taken as the highest dilution of the serum which gives a positive result. The density of the floccules may be indicated by the number of pluses given against the result.

The *V.D.R.L.* test, devised by the Reference Laboratory (U.S.), is a similar type of test and is also widely used.

Specific Treponemal Tests

These consist of test procedures using a treponemal antigen, and include the following:—

REITER'S PROTEIN COMPLEMENT FIXATION TEST (RPCFT)

The technique of this test is essentially that of the W.R. Lyophilized Reiter protein antigen (avirulent treponeme) is commercially available.

TREPONEMA PALLIDUM IMMOBILIZATION (TPI)

This test owing to its complexity is performed in special laboratories. The antigen consists of live treponemes (virulent Nichol strain) obtained from a rabbit testicular syphiloma. Inactivated serum, complement and a suspension of treponemes are mixed together, incubated anaerobically at 35° C. for 18 hours, and examined under dark-ground microscopy. 'Immobilization' of the treponemes in the test-tubes must be compared with treponemal motility in a control tube.

FLUORESCENT TREPONEMAL ANTIBODY (FTA) TEST

The FTA test is more accurate when accompanied by an absorption procedure, which removes the bulk of the cross-reacting non-specific treponemal antibody, known as the *FTA-ABS* test.

Reagents required are: a suspension of Nichol's strain treponemes from rabbit syphiloma; conjugate: fluorescein-labelled antihuman globulin (rabbit) serum; buffered saline (pH 7·2) and glycerin for mounting; inactivated human serum.

Principle of method: 0·01 ml. of treponemal suspension is placed on a slide, dried in the air, and fixed in acetone for 10 minutes; 0·03 ml. of a 1 : 200 dilution of human serum in buffered saline is added, and the mixture incubated in a moist atmosphere at 37° C. for one hour; it is then washed in two changes of buffered saline for five minutes. Dilute conjugate 0·03 ml. (for titres) is incubated at moist 37° C. for half an hour; then washed in buffered saline as before. The sample is mounted in a drop of buffered saline (one part) and glycerin (nine parts), and examined with dark-ground condenser in the dark, using ultra-violet light source and filter transmitting radiations 2500–3900 Å. A positive fluorescence, using fluorescent dye, is indicated by a brilliant green colour. Control sera, both positive and negative, are included in all tests.

Dark-ground Oil Immersion Microscopy and Collection of Specimens

See Chapter 2 (Early Infectious Syphilis—Chancre), p. 21.

CHAPTER 14

Antibiotics in Venereal Disease

The term 'antibiotic' has been used for many antibacterial agents, dating from the time of the discovery of penicillin: the sulphonamides and other so-called chemotherapeutic agents are excluded. The word is not a very good one since it refers more precisely to something which is antagonistic to all life.

The majority of antibiotics in use have been developed originally from natural sources. They act upon one or more of three basic areas of structure or function in the micro-organism: the wall, the protoplast membrane, or the nucleic acid and protein synthesis. Differences in these areas, between one micro-organism and another, are responsible for the differing activities of the many antibiotics.

The staining properties of bacteria, for example, are related to their structures. Thus Gram-negative bacteria have walls containing many amino acids and a high lipid content. Gram-positive ones have little lipid and few amino acids; but the cell wall of Gram-positive bacteria has an outer layer, separable from the underlying lipoprotein membrane, and has no enzyme activity. Antibiotics acting on (1) the wall are penicillins, cephalosporins, vancomycin, novobiocin, etc. (2) The protoplast membrane, which acts as an osmotic barrier, as well as being a site for the synthesis of certain cell constituents, is affected by streptomycin, tyrocidin, gramicidin, polymyxin and novobiocin. (3) Nucleic acid and protein synthesis is interfered with by the tetracyclines, streptomycin and chloramphenicol. The first two groups of antibiotic drugs mentioned are mainly *bactericidal*, and the last group mainly *bacteriostatic*. They are active in the presence of pus, and reach all tissues in the body; their concentrations in the cerebrospinal fluid, however, are lower than in the blood. But since neurological disorder in syphilis, for example, is almost entirely mediated *via* the blood vessels, circulating antibiotic usually reaches lesions in the nervous system in this way.

Owing to their effectiveness and lack of side-effects in many instances, these drugs have tended to be used indiscriminately, either before diagnosis or for trivial infection. This is to be regretted for several reasons, and especially in the context of the sexually transmitted diseases: firstly it confuses the diagnosis and suppresses rather than cures disease; secondly it encourages the emergence of insensitive strains of micro-organism.

PENICILLIN

This was the first antibiotic to be isolated. It is relatively non-toxic. *Penicillin G (benzyl)* is the most active species; it is inactivated by the gastric juice and has to be given by injection. *Penicillin V (phenoxymethyl)* is stable as an acid, and can be taken by mouth. The semisynthetic *phenethicillin* and *ampicillin* can also be taken orally: alone of these, ampicillin has a broad spectrum of activity. Cloxacillin is unaffected by penicillinase.

The naturally occurring penicillins do not inhibit Gram-negative bacilli nor penicillinase-producing staphylococci; both characteristics possessed by ampicillin and the latter alone by cloxacillin. They are active, however, against other types of staphylococci, streptococci, pneumococci and other Gram-negative bacteria; also against gonococci, as well as certain other organisms such as the spirochaetes, including Vincent's spirillum and all treponemes. They are chiefly used in the present context in the treatment of syphilis and gonorrhoea.

Penicillin acts by inhibiting mucopeptide synthesis in the cell wall. Over half the amount taken by the patient can be recovered in the urine: this excretion can be slowed and the blood levels raised by giving *probenecid* 1·0 g. daily by mouth. Following an intramuscular injection of benzylpenicillin in watery solution, of whatever quantity, there are only minimal amounts remaining in the blood after four hours. *With procaine penicillin G*, there are significant levels after 12 and even 18 hours, and with *benzathine penicillin*, after several days.

Side effects include (1) immediate: urticaria, angio-neurotic oedema and anaphylactic shock, (2) intermediate (hours to two days): oedema, wheals and fever, (3) delayed (days to three weeks): papulo-vesicular rash, pruritus, fever, arthralgia; or dermatitis, purpura, angiitis, and an Arthus phenomenon. The method of treatment varies with the kind and the severity of the reaction and should include: lying the patient flat, 0·5–1·0 ml. subcutaneous or intramuscular injection of 1 : 1000 adrenaline hydrochloride, intramuscular antihistamine drug (chlorphenira-mine 10–20 mg.) or hydrocortisone 20–50 mg. repeated, and given intravenously if necessary.

In the treatment of early syphilis a form of therapeutic reaction or shock occurs, manifested by fever and malaise, the Jarisch-Herxheimer reaction. No special treatment is required. Prophy-laxis consists in administering prednisolone 20 mg. by mouth for a few days prior to the onset of treatment (see Treatment of Syphilis p. 70).

CEPHALOSPORIN C

This is related to penicillin. It has a lower toxicity than penicillin, and no cross-hypersensitivity with penicillin occurs. Being poorly absorbed from the intestine, however, it has to be given by intramuscular injection in doses of 0·5–1 g. every six hours, or 2·0 g. in one injection daily. It is useful where there is hyper-sensitivity to penicillin.

STREPTOMYCIN

Other members of this group are *dihydrostreptomycin*, *neomycin*, *kanamycin* and *viomycin*. Streptomycin was discovered soon after penicillin. It is active against Gram-negative bacteria, Gram-positive enterococci and the tubercle bacillus. It is useful therefore in renal tract infections and in gonorrhoea; although in the latter, as in other infections, insensitive strains soon arise.

Unlike penicillin streptomycin is not destroyed by the bacteria. It is bacteriostatic and bactericidal and acts by damage to the cell membrane and interference with protein synthesis.

Adverse effects of the drug are manifested by giddiness, tinnitus and impairment of hearing (due to VIII cranial nerve damage), and by an immediate sense of tightening and heat about the face. Other effects are: fever, vomiting and skin reactions, and it is unwise to use the drug in cases of renal damage except when due to tuberculosis. Streptomycin is not readily absorbed from the gut and has therefore to be given by intramuscular injection in doses of 0·5–1·0 g., dissolved in distilled water, once or twice daily. For enteritis the drug may be given by mouth. If the drug is given by mouth, vitamin supplements of B complex and K are necessary.

Treatment of lower genito-urinary inflammation including gonorrhoea and other forms of urethritis, with streptomycin, is useful when a coexistent syphilitic infection is suspected since the treponeme is not affected by the usual dose of this drug. It may also be used in granuloma inguinale and chancroid.

TETRACYCLINE

This group consists of several related compounds having similar properties, *tetracycline*, *oxytetracycline*, *chlortetracycline*, *methacycline*, and *demethylchlortetracycline*. A proportion of the tetracycline is rapidly absorbed from the stomach and small intestine, and mainly excreted by the kidneys. The principal side-effects arise from intestinal irritation mainly due to a changed intestinal flora. The commonest is pruritus ani and vulvae. Nausea and diarrhoea can occur; rashes are uncommon. Growth of candida in the alimentary tract follows their prolonged use. Hypoplasia, and staining of the enamel of the teeth has occurred with their use in young children, and their use in pregnancy is not desirable. Degradation products in old and badly stored tetracycline may result in renal damage.

The tetracyclines have a wide range of activity, against Gram-positive and Gram-negative bacteria, treponemes, and smaller organisms such as mycoplasma and the Chlamydia group of large viruses.

The drug is therefore of use in most of the infective causes of lower genito-urinary disease, which are described in the foregoing pages. It takes second place to penicillin in the treatment of syphilis and gonorrhoea, It is the drug of choice for abacterial and non-trichomonal urethritis, and lymphogranuloma venereum.

Tetracycline is given orally in the usual dose of 0·25 g. every six hours. Chlortetracycline and oxytetracycline are used in the same manner.

ERYTHROMYCIN

This antibiotic can be given orally and is effective against certain Gram-positive bacteria, Neisseria, and treponemes. Its action is mainly bacteriostatic. It is related in structure to oleandomycin, spiramycin and carbomycin. It is not so dependable, however, for the treatment of syphilis. It is relatively free from side-effects; but nausea and diarrhoea may follow the use of the drug in excess of 0·25–0·5 g. six-hourly.

CHLORAMPHENICOL

The use of chloramphenicol is restricted owing to a toxic action on the bone marrow. This complication is a rare one, but almost always fatal. The drug is rapidly absorbed from the gastro-intestinal tract, and, like the tetracyclines, has a wide range of activity. It is useful for local application (half per cent solution) on the skin, and in the eye or the nose. It is given to stubborn infections of the renal tract, Haemophilus, Brucella and Salmonella infections, in doses of 0·25 g. six-hourly.

Spiramycin, Carbomycin, Oleandomycin, Vancomycin, Novobiocin, Bacitracin, Albamycin, Lincomycin

These amongst others, also have their place as antibacterial agents. But they are of less importance than those already described.

Tyrothricin (a mixture of gramicidin and tryocidin) is used as a local application, 0·5 mg./ml. as an isotonic solution. Local reactions are uncommon. It is effective against Gram-positive organisms.

Polymyxin B is limited to intravenous and to local use; *Polymyxin E* can be given intramuscularly, being active against Gram-negative organisms, though not against proteus. It is used in strengths of 0·1–1·0 per cent aqueous solution or ointment. Parenterally the drug can result in renal and nerve damage.

Nystatin is active against several yeasts and moulds: but its clinical usefulness is limited to mycotic infections caused by candida. It is fungistatic and fungicidal, and applied in a pessary or suppository containing 100,000 units. It is relatively insoluble in water, and not absorbed from the alimentary tract.

Amphotericin B is fungistatic. Both this drug and nystatin act by damaging the protoplasmic membrane of the fungi. Amphotericin has a broad spectrum of antifungal activity. Since it is not absorbed, it must be given intravenously, 0·25 mg./kg. body weight. The drug is slowly excreted by the kidney. Reactions include headache and fever, and occasionally a rise in blood urea, the renal damage being reversible. It is successfully used as a local application in candida infections.

Griseofulvin, because of its affinity for keratin, is effective against superficial infections of hair, skin and nails caused by the epidermophyton, trichophyton and microsporon species. It is of little value against candida. It is given orally, 0·25 g. six-hourly. Side-effects include gastro-intestinal symptoms, headache, neurological features and skin rashes.

Antibiotic and Chemotherapeutic Combinations

A combination of two antibiotics resulting in an *antagonism* or lessening of the effect which either one would have if given alone, can occur. This antagonism has been recorded in a clinical setting when penicillin and tetracycline, and penicillin and chloramphenicol have been used together, and there is some experimental evidence to support it. Thus there is a guiding rule that a bactericidal drug has little chance of acting if used in the presence of a bacteriostatic one. Theoretically this is an important consideration, but evidence until recently has been small, and in practice each case has had to be judged on its merits. Tetracycline, chloramphenicol and erythromycin may partly or wholly antagonise the bactericidal action of the penicillins, cephalosporins and vancomycin.

The existence of a *potentiation*, that is, of more than a simple additive effect when using two antibiotic drugs at once, is clinically demonstrable. Such a potentiating effect results when penicillin and streptomycin are given together. This has also been noted when penicillin or cephalosporin is combined with kanamycin; and when streptomycin and tetracycline are used together in brucellosis. There is evidence, too, for this potentiation in the sphere of chemotherapeutic agents: for example, trimethoprim plus sulphamethoxazole.

Antibiotics of Choice in Venereal Disease

In *syphilis* penicillin by injection remains the drug of choice. Tetracycline by mouth, and cephalosporin by injection are the next most useful, probably in this order with tetracycline being the most dependable. Erythromycin may be tried.

For *lymphogranuloma venereum*, *granuloma inguinale* and *chancroid*, the tetracyclines may be used. However, when syphilis is suspected, sulphonamides should be exhibited in lymphogranuloma venereum, and streptomycin in the other two conditions.

Gonorrhoea is treated in many countries primarily with penicillin, either by injection or in children with an oral preparation. Tetracycline is the next drug of choice; although the organism is sensitive to a large number of antibiotics in general use, any of which, such as erythromycin, may be used in sufficient dosage.

Abacterial urethritis, excluding that due to thrush or trichomonas, is best treated with tetracycline in the first instance. Specific causes such as the trichomonas are treated with the requisite drug as described.

SELECTED BIBLIOGRAPHY FOR ANTIBIOTICS IN VENEREAL DISEASE

PENICILLIN REACTIONS

Idsoe, I., Guthie, T., Willcox, R. R. & De Weck, A. L. (1968). *Bull. Wld Hlth Org.* **38**, 159.

ANTIBIOTIC AND CHEMOTHERAPEUTIC COMBINATIONS

Manten, A. & Terra, J. I. (1964). *Chemotherapia*, **8**, 21.

Manten, A. (1967). In *Proceedings of 5th International Congress* Stuttgart: Georg Thieme.

INDEX

PRINTED BY NEILL & CO. LTD., 212 CAUSEWAYSIDE, EDINBURGH